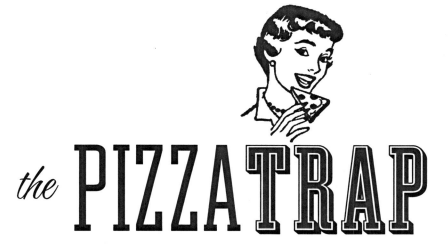

the PIZZA TRAP

EVERY MOM'S GUIDE TO
BREAKING CHILDREN'S DANGEROUS FOOD ADDICTIONS,
ENDING MEALTIME BATTLES AND
BUILDING HEALTHY HABITS FOR LIFE

Gabrielle Welch

NC, CHHC

WITH FOREWORD BY DEVINDER BHATIA, MD

Front Cover Design By:
Allyson Lack, Principle
www.designbyprinciple.com

Book design by Kerrie Lian under contract with MacGraphics Services: www.MacGraphics.net

Gabrielle Welch
Visit my website at www.WelchWellness.com; www.The PizzaTrap.com

Printed in the United States of America

First Printing: December 2012

ISBN-13: 978-0-9859069-0-0 (paperback)
eISBN: 978-0-9859069-1-7 (e-book)
LCCN: 2012920154

The author and publisher endeavors to make the information in this book accurate and up to date. It is a general guide. Before taking action on significant medical, legal or financial matters you should consult with qualified professionals who can help you consider your unique circumstances. The author and publisher cannot accordingly accept any liability for any loss or damage suffered as a consequence of relying on the information contained in this book.

Mention of specific leaders in research, education, marriage and family therapy, or other authorities in this book does not imply they endorse this book. Internet addresses are accurate at the time of printing.

*The book is dedicated to my mother, Ethel,
and husband Rallin, who made it all possible.*

In loving memory of my brother Patrick.

Contents

Foreword

When I first decided to enter into the field of medicine, I was no older than the children we are writing about in this book. I imagined myself performing lifesaving surgeries on older adults, but little did I know that one day I would be operating on the younger generations as well.

Today, there is a dramatic increase in the development of diabetes, hypertension and early onset coronary artery disease in young Americans. With one third of the country's children considered obese, it's no wonder that such diseases are becoming more and more prevalent. In less than ten years approximately 30 percent of children ages eight to ten will become diabetic and/or hypertensive.

A sedentary lifestyle certainly contributes to the increase in these diseases. Our kids rarely go outside and play. The basketball court and baseball diamonds have been replaced with Wii and Play Stations. But in addition to a less active lifestyle, poor diets are a major contributor to the development of adult diseases in our children.

Currently, it seems to be more challenging than ever for parents to expose their children to healthy food. Busier households, often with two working parents, lead to night after night of fast-food and quick and easy snacking. These processed junk foods contain more saturated fats than ever before. And they appeal to us—and our kids—because we have conditioned ourselves to eat these foods on a daily basis.

Even as the media continues to discuss the dangers of unhealthy eating, it appears that we are going in the wrong direction. Instead of quarter pounders, we now have half pounders. Instead of half-sizing fast foods, we double size them. Even in situations where "good" foods are served, the portion sizes have increased across the board.

As more and more children develop diseases linked to unhealthy eating, like early onset coronary artery disease, hypertension and diabetes —diabetes can lead to peripheral vascular disease, kidney failure, blindness, coronary disease and premature death—our health care system will face an unimaginable burden. Doctors and health care facilities will be unnaturally taxed and the cost to treat these young patients may lead to fiscal mayhem.

The day I performed heart surgery on someone my own age was a wakeup call. The day I operated on someone younger than me was bone chilling. I never imagined that I would be operating on kids with adult-acquired diseases. Yes, things are bad, but thankfully they're not hopeless. After reading *The Pizza Trap* I wholeheartedly recommend and endorse it. Gabrielle Welch clearly and decisively outlines ways in which parents and other caregivers can apply the brakes to the runaway train of unhealthy eating and put their kids on a path to lifelong health and wellness. It is essential to address the way our kids eat today.

—Dr. Devinder Bhatia

"Be the change you wish to see in the world."

— GANDHI

We live in a fast-food, junk-food, fake-food world. Quick and easy processed foods are everywhere. Each day, our little ones are bombarded with the temptation to eat foods that are instantly gratifying yet dangerously low in nutritional value. Junk food has become a national bad habit, one that is turning our kids into terrifying statistics. As our children get further away from whole foods and deeper into the seemingly unending cycle of sweet and salty processed foods, the prevalence of childhood food allergies is steadily on the rise[1] and 17 percent of American children are obese.[2] Our children are also experiencing significant increases in autism,[3] asthma,[4] and ADHD[5]— three conditions that have been linked to obesity, poor nutrition, processed foods and food additives.

Eating a balanced diet—low in saturated fats and sugars and high in whole grains, vegetables and lean meats—has been proven to dramatically benefit the long-term health of our kids. Yet few parents feel equipped to guide their children down a path of healthy eating. As a mom of three young kids, I can relate. Instilling healthy eating habits in my kids once seemed like an impossible task—especially because junk food is everywhere.

Junk food is now a category that encompasses more than salty snacks and sweet treats. Severely unhealthy fare has wiggled its way into mainstream eating, masquerading as legitimate options for breakfast, lunch and dinner. Here's an example of a typical American child's daily menu:

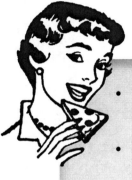

- **Muffins, kolaches or donuts in the morning:** these baked goods are loaded with sugar and trans fat.
- **Peanut butter and jelly for lunch:** most peanuts are harvested with pesticides and/or herbicides, combined with partially hydrogenated oil and excessive salt; jelly made with pesticide-coated fruit, processed sugar and artificial color; white bread containing bleached flour, genetically modified soybean oil plus lecithin and corn syrup.
- **Macaroni and cheese, a hot dog or pizza for dinner:** dough and cheese made with processed white flour, yellow dye #5 and #6, high sodium, MSG and artificial flavors; hot dogs loaded with nitrites, high fructose corn syrup, MSG and artificial flavors.

These foods, loaded with sugars, salts and fats are highly addictive—our kids crave them consistently. Yet when we succumb to our children's cravings, when we give in to their nagging, their whining—the begging and pleading that happens every time you drive past a fast-food restaurant or stroll past the food court in the mall or pause in front of your own refrigerator at night—we are caught in the trap. Anytime we replace whole, real foods with an easier option, we have been snagged in what I call the Pizza Trap.

Recently, Grant Hill, a famous NBA player with the Phoenix Suns, said that he remembered his mom naming pizza as one of the "best foods" because it contains all of the major food groups. Hill's mother is not alone. Many parents believe that pizza and many other highly processed junk foods are healthy options for their kids.

While the combination of flour, tomato sauce and cheese may be easy and tasty, it is anything but healthy. Pizza is full of fat, sodium, sugar and typically packed with harmful flavor-enhancing preservatives. Yet at most birthday parties, sleepovers and school events, pizza is the food that's most commonly served. Pizza is even a staple in school cafeterias—a menu option now protected by Congress, which officially declared the food a "vegetable."

One slice of pizza with a side salad and fruit is okay occasionally. But how many kids stop at one slice? And how often is a salad served with it? More often than not, pizza is paired with sodas or sugary energy drinks, with cake and ice cream for dessert. Later in the guide, I'll offer some healthier alternatives to take-out pizza and will let you know what exactly is going into your kids' bodies when they eat a pizzeria slice.

Changing the way your kids relate to pizza—and other unhealthy foods—is possible. I know this because I live it. As a nutritional consultant, I see my clients struggling to offer their children a well-balanced diet. And as a mom, every day (at least three times a day) I face the task of educating my family about the value of eating whole, real foods. Junk food has a very real hold on our kids, but ultimately we make the rules.

It's true, we're working against a lot. Parents have to see past the kids' menu at restaurants and the offerings at the school cafeteria. We have to push against a billion dollar marketing machine that feeds nonstop TV advertising campaigns and blockbuster product placements. We have to stand up to friends and neighbors and family members who placate and reward with junk food.

Here's the good news: even amidst the onslaught of social pressure, you hold the power to change the way your kids eat. You control your child's lunch box and what ends up on their dinner plate each night. You buy the groceries. You prepare the food. By setting a positive example (what are *your* food choices?) and empowering kids with knowledge about where their food comes from, you have the opportunity to cultivate healthy habits in the next generation and beyond.

The Pizza Trap is not about counting calories, fat grams or sodium. We've all had enough of that. Instead, this guide offers effective tips for putting an end to mealtime food battles and dangerous food addictions. Pulling from my own experiences at the dinner table and years as a nutritional consultant working closely with parents, I offer simple solutions for real families living in a junk food world.

Now is the time to start.

Why Now?

The declining health of American children—and of children in countries where the US food industry has a growing presence—is an indicator that something is horribly wrong with how our young ones are eating. As I listen to the concerns of parents who seek out my services as a nutritional consultant and watch what's going on in my own children's world, I realize what a true epidemic we are facing. As a mother, trying to help my kids build lifelong healthy eating habits in a society that pushes quite the opposite, I face the same daily challenges you do.

We fight for the lives of our children when we fight against the Standard American Diet (SAD), which consists of highly refined and processed foods and sugary drinks. All children are subject to and influenced by the Big Food marketing machine, made up of monopolies that dominate the food system and the government. Big Food marketing is everywhere and often promotes products targeted directly to kids and teens. For example, spending to promote child-targeted cereals was $264 million in 2011, an increase of more than 30 percent from 2008.[1]

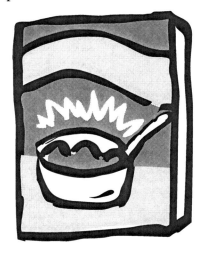

I have seen the real-life impact that Big Food culture has on our children. I have worked with overweight kids who suffer from cholesterol and heart issues that were at one time solely adult conditions. I have clients whose kids won't eat anything but a handful of white processed foods—pasta, bread, chicken nuggets and the like. After years of consuming these sometimes bland, sometimes overly salty and definitely nutritionally empty foods, whole foods like broccoli or even an apple smell and taste unpleasant to them—resulting in eating habits that lead to significant vitamin deficiency.

Here's a look at some startling statistics that reveal the effects that junk food and sedentary lifestyles are having on our children.

- *This is the first generation of children that is not expected to outlive their parents.[2]*

- *One in three kids born in the year 2000 is expected to be diabetic by the time he or she reaches adulthood.[3]*

- *As a nation, we consume 140–200 lbs. of sugar annually.[4] The prevalence of obesity in US children has quadrupled since the 1960's and 32 percent of American kids between the ages of two and nineteen are overweight—and this number is growing daily. Half of these kids are obese.[5]*

- *According to the Henry J. Kaiser Foundation, children ages eight to eighteen spend 7.5 hours in front of a screen daily— this includes television, computer and video games. Excessive screen time is one of many causes of rising obesity statistics in children.*

- *Today, it is estimated that 20 percent of American children have allergies. An allergy is an overreaction of the immune system that can affect any system of the body, including respiratory, cardiovascular, gastrointestinal and epidermal. Many popular foods in the United States contain chemicals and toxins that have been linked to alarming increases in childhood allergies as well as ADHD, cancer and asthma.[6]*

THE ASTHMA EPIDEMIC

In the last twenty years, we have seen an epidemic increase in allergies, asthma, ADHD and autism, including

- 400 percent increase in food allergies;

- 300 percent increase in asthma, with a 56 percent increase in asthma deaths;

- 400 percent increase in ADHD; and

- between a 1,500 and 6,000 percent increase in autism.

The male/female ratio for food allergies is 2:1 and the male/female ratio for asthma is 3:1.[7]

"*Healthy citizens are the greatest asset any country can have.*"

—WINSTON CHURCHILL

How Schools Fail Our Kids

Whether we put our children on the bus in the morning or drop them off at school, we trust that academically they will be taught what they need to know to succeed in life. But school is not only about academic instruction. School is for socialization and learning life lessons as well.

Schools teach children how to protect themselves from bullies. They teach them about body safety and stranger danger. They teach them how to "just say no" to drugs, alcohol and sex. But when it comes to food, our schools fail miserably in educating our kids about healthy eating and providing nutritious options at lunchtime.

America is now facing an epidemic of overfed and undernourished kids who spend most of their time in front of a screen. These children live on junk food, are disconnected from nature, watch over 40,000 commercials on TV each year[8] and get almost no exercise. And most schools do very little to instill healthy eating habits in children. Across the board, school lunches in our country are severely lacking in nutrition, quality and variety. As a nutritional consultant and mom, when I walk through a hot lunch line and see fried chicken tenders, tater tots and canned green beans that aren't green (and by the way aren't being eaten by the kids because they have no flavor) being served for lunch, my heart breaks.

Although activists like Jamie Oliver and his Food Revolution have made a genuine effort to inform schools, kids and parents about nutrition, we still have a long way to go.

As parents we have a responsibility to advocate for healthy school lunches. Many schools offer "lunch and learn" programs for the parents on the topic of nutrition, but what we learn about nutrition we are unable to teach or enforce because healthy lunch choices are not being provided by the school. Schools have budgetary restrictions, which often limit their ability to provide healthy food options. This is where community organizing and activism can make a difference. Schools and governments respond to the organized and methodically communicated concern of parents and the community. I have seen concerned parents work miracles over time: organic gardens have been planted by children and the vegetables have been harvested and cooked at the school. Vending machines selling junk food have been outlawed in several school districts across the nation and vending machines companies, like Sprout Healthy Vending (www.sprouthealthyvending.com), that offer healthy drinks, snacks, yogurt and smoothies have taken their place!

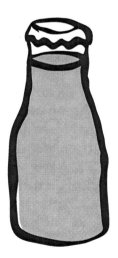

Thelunchtray.com, fedupwithlunch. com and thelunchbox.org are wonderful blogs and resources where parents can stay in touch with the most recent food issues and topics facing our nation, our children and our schools. Looking for fun, healthy and creative lunch ideas for your kids? Take a look at meetthedubiens.com, crafty moods.com, and cometogetherkidsblogspot.com for some very inspiring lunches from some highly creative moms.

These incredible women have taken it to the next level with their creative and fun approach to food and crafts. If you're feeling blah, tired of making the same lunches and snacks every day, or are trying to inspire your child, these sites are great resources.

Another school-related factor that contributes to the rise in obesity and general ill-health of our kids is the national cut back on physical education. Many public schools have limited PE to one day a week, even in affluent neighborhoods. Schools are sacrificing recess and PE to give kids more "class time," often so that they can win acclaims on their math and English testing to keep their standing as a nationally or statewide recognized public school. What price are our kids paying with their health?

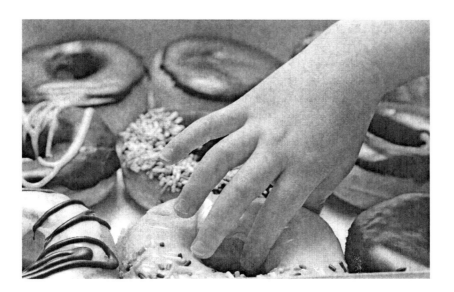

Rethinking Birthday Cupcakes

SIGH. If I had a dollar for every time one of my girls came home and said they had donut holes at recess I would be a very wealthy woman. Instead, I have been a frustrated mom looking for alternatives to the excessive treats they get every time someone has a birthday at school, which in my opinion is way too often. At the same time, like every other parent, I want my girls to celebrate and have fun with their school friends.

Do you want your children indulging in donut holes, brownies, cookies or a cupcake in the middle of the school day, several days a week (I swear it's that often)? Especially after they have already had chocolate milk and a dessert at lunch? Do you know what it does to their ability to focus in school and perform athletically? Even worse, with all those daytime sugary treats, kids may still request a snack from the concession stand after softball practice and dessert after dinner at home. You can break the sugar cycle with creative alternatives to birthday sweets that kids actually love. Get creative! Rewards or treats don't always have to be about food. Take a trip to the dollar store with your child and let them choose something for their classmates. Or better yet, find a fun craft they can work on at home to share with their classmates. There are some great ideas out there on the internet, like having a butterfly release for the kids: each child gets a caterpillar and the class watches them grow until release time. Chocolate dipped pretzels or strawberries are a great choice for a birthday treat, as is decorating a T- shirt for the birthday boy or girl with fabric markers (Visit the lunchtray.com for more great ideas). The upside to this also is that kids with food allergies can participate as well. If you believe that your child is getting too much sugar during the day, don't be afraid to take a stand and make a change. No one else is going to do it for you, and you might be surprised to find out how many other parents, and possibly your school, feel the same way. You might get some initial push back from your child, but you can handle it! If they insist on bringing a treat, homemade options are always healthier (and less expensive) than store bought. You can also make dietary adjustments if necessary for those that have allergies, dairy or gluten sensitivities.

DOES YOUR CHILD HAVE NATURE DEFICIT DISORDER?

Less PE and more time in front of screens not only contributes to the growing childhood obesity epidemic but now, as parents, we have something else to look out for: the growing national problem of Nature Deficit Disorder. A term coined by Richard

Louv in his 2005 book *Last Child in the Woods*, Nature Deficit Disorder refers to the increasing amount of time that children spend indoors, disconnected from nature. According to Louv, this lack of time with the natural world results in a wide range of behavioral problems including depression, hyperactivity, shorter attention span and obesity.

New research shows that 19 percent of children ages two to five know how to use a Smartphone, but only 9 percent can tie their shoes, and more children know how to play a computer game than ride a bike (www.youroutdoorfamily.com, "Nature Deficit Disorder Alive and Well," Jenny Veal, February 1, 2011).

Kids are meant to be outside, not only to exercise and receive their daily dose of vitamin D—which may help prevent depression and other diseases—but to be with and learn about nature while laughing and engaging in healthy social activities. Make sure that your children are getting as much time outdoors as possible. If it's hard to accomplish during the week, make a special effort on weekends to get them outside in the sunshine moving their bodies as much as possible. Trade off with a friend every other week if it's too hard to accomplish on your own.

You *Become* What You Eat

With consistency, your kids will begin to see the connection between the foods they eat and their energy levels, overall health and sleeping patterns. They may also begin to see a correlation between how well they do in school and how happy they feel when they are consistently eating whole, real foods. Take a recent client of mine, Matt. As an eight-year-old diagnosed with ADHD, Matt suffered from behavioral challenges that made it difficult for him to focus in school or engage with other children—uncontrollable tantrums and angry outbursts were part of his everyday life. However, when Matt's mom cleaned out the pantry and stopped buying food with artificial coloring and additives Matt's behavior began to improve. Several weeks later, at his school's field day he chose to have a red and blue sno-cone. Within thirty minutes, he spiraled out of control: yelling, screaming, crying and lashing out at those around him. After he was able to calm down hours later, Matt's mom explained the connection to him, and he immediately understood. He then personally made the choice to avoid trigger foods. Now, every time I see him he runs up to me proudly and tells me how great he is feeling with less artificially flavored and colored food in his diet.

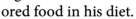

We made the decision to bring our kids into this world and it is our responsibility to teach them how to make good decisions for themselves while we still have them at home. We get eighteen years to provide our children with the life skills they need to survive outside the nest; this includes learning how to care for their bodies. It is our role as parents to teach them to question what's put in front of them—whether it's a cigarette, alcohol or a hot dog—and to trust their gut, both literally and figuratively. We are the ones who will introduce our children to the connection between what they eat and how good they feel.

"Let food be thy medicine, and thy medicine be food."

—HIPPOCRATES

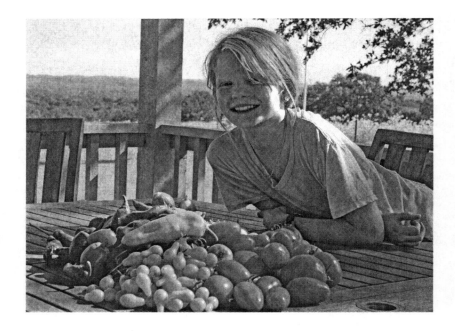

Reconnecting to the Source of Our Food

Do peaches and carrots and ground beef magically appear on supermarket shelves? Where does the food we eat come from? These questions take on greater importance as we have become increasingly disconnected from the source of our food. When your child eats something, does she understand that it originally came out of the ground from a seed or that it was recently a living, breathing animal? Sadly, many children are so removed from where their food comes from that they don't associate the chicken that they eat with the chicken in the farmyard or the French fry with a potato.

Most children have never been to a farm or even a farmers market for that matter. Many don't know what a food co-op is, especially those growing up in large cities. And very few children

Kids often associate vegetables with the ones they see on fast-food sandwiches: white, tasteless lettuce and an under ripe or over-ripe tomato. I don't like those vegetables either. They have no flavor and no nutrients. Make an effort to find ripe, organic fruits and vegetables for your children and they will begin to associate produce with fresh and exciting flavor. Look for SKU numbers on fruits and veggies that begin with a 9: these indicate organic, non-genetically modified choices.

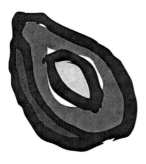

have had the opportunity to plant a seed, watch it grow, harvest and eat the result. And how many children are lucky enough to have seen an actual chicken lay an egg and pick it up while it's still warm to the touch? How many kids have had the experience of picking a juicy, ripe red tomato right off the vine and biting into it as is—free from pesticides, herbicides or chemicals? How many have tasted raw milk from a cow?

I had a five-year-old child recently look at me like I was crazy when I told him that the baked chicken we were having for dinner was actually chicken. He had never seen it in any other form than a nugget. In fact, my own six-year-old refused to believe that a hamburger actually came from one of the pretty cows she sees walking around her grandmother's ranch. A child has even asked me if there is such a thing as a "Cheetos tree."

Most children in our country go to the supermarket with their mom, dad or grandparents and pick perfectly prepackaged foods off the shelf: beef, chicken, pork, eggs and milk on the perimeter of the store and the dreaded snack food and junk items in the center aisles. How can they possibly comprehend what went in to making those foods? It's our responsibility to teach our kids the difference between real food and fake food. Fake food has been highly altered and processed to make it taste good. We must educate our children about the difference between whole foods and processed foods. Studying labels together is a great way to start. The nacho-cheese-flavored tortilla chips made with eighteen ingredients—some of them unpronounceable—are not a healthy option. While celery sticks dipped in peanut butter—two ingredients: peanuts and salt—are a wonderful choice. If you pick a ripe apple or orange off a tree, do you need to change anything to make it taste good? Consistently offering your kids healthy options will help them understand that real food tastes good on its own: it doesn't need help.

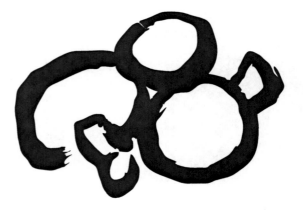

Many mothers of two- to five-year-old kids come to me and say, "I don't understand what's happened. As a baby he ate all the jarred fruits, veggies and proteins I served him. There was nothing he wouldn't eat. Now, he only eats four or five things: fries, chicken nuggets, hot dogs and pasta or white bread. What happened?" What happened is that these parents slowly got sucked into what I call the "New Normal"—cheap, easy and fast food that doesn't include anything green. The kind of food that lives at the ballpark, movie theater, concession stand, in the freezer, and on the kids' menu almost everywhere you go.

Don't become a victim of this New Normal. As soon as your child begins transitioning to real foods, make sure to continue feeding them a variety of fruits and veggies with every meal, no matter where you are, even if it necessitates bringing supplies with you to a restaurant or sports field. No time to shop? Frozen veggies can live in the freezer next to the chicken tenders and tater tots, too, and are a great alternative to fresh ones. My kids love to eat frozen green beans!

Food as Big Business

It is not only our children who are misinformed about where our food comes from. Many times, we are just as disconnected as they are. We may know that a hamburger comes from a cow or a nugget comes from a chicken, but do we know where that cow came from? Do we know what it was fed or how it was raised and treated? The answers to these questions are very important when choosing what food to eat.

It is by design that we are so disconnected from the source of our food supply. If we really knew where our food was coming from, and what was in it, we would be shocked. The advances of industrialized agriculture have contributed significantly to the rise of the major businesses that hold so much control over the food system in today's society. Until we dig in and discover the truth

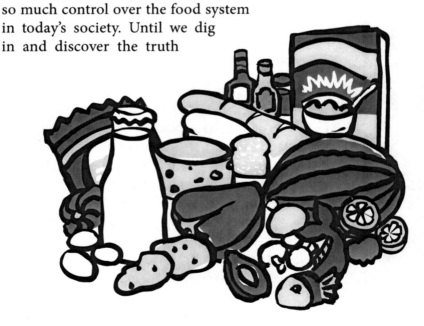

about our food chain here in the United States, they will continue to hold the power and we will continue to get sicker.

Food is big business in our nation. Why else are we still fighting to eliminate GM (genetically modified) foods from our food supply—or at least have them labeled—and to remove artificial food dyes from our foods, when a large number of other industrialized nations did it years ago? Many large companies, like Sam's Club, were fast to comply, removing the toxic ingredients from their products in Europe because of the large consumer demand. If they can do it there, why don't we do it here? The answer lies in the fact that corporate profit is the primary motivation of our food suppliers, not concern for our children's health. Did you know that the profit margin for soft drinks is 90 percent, while the profit seen from fruit and veggie sales is about 10 percent?[9]

> This is the first generation of children who are NOT EXPECTED TO OUTLIVE THEIR PARENTS! How did we get here? How is this possible?

FDA AND LARGE FOOD CORPORATIONS— THE REVOLVING DOOR

It's natural to assume that the Food and Drug Administration is looking after our children's health, but in reality employees are flip-flopping constantly between the FDA and the food and chemical companies that refuse to change their policies to keep our kids safe. For example, someone from a cereal company that sells sugary, unhealthy breakfast food to our kids may acquire a new position in the FDA. So now, that person is making binding decisions about what's good or bad for our children when their entire career has been focused on selling sugary cereal to kids! This is an eye-opener that we can't count on something being good for our kids simply because it is "FDA approved."

As parents, we also need to be aware of the motivation behind the ad campaigns that we see every day on billboards, TV and at the grocery store. Their goal is not to keep our kids' healthy, it's to make money. Period. The milk and beef industries have some of the most pervasive—and persuasive—campaigns and target directly to parents, using fear and our ignorance to sell their products.

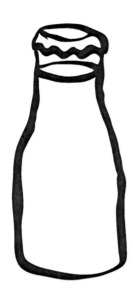

Got Milk?

We have all been told from a very early age that milk is essential to our health. As a result of all the great advertising as well as the push from pediatricians, the US Dairy Industry produced over $20 billion in sales in 2002.[10]

I, too, encouraged my children (at least the first two) to drink as much milk as possible, believing that I was doing the right thing. At my urging, my oldest two children had "milk races" to see who could drink the most milk each day (reliving this is not a proud moment for me). I then reported my oldest daughter's milk consumption (five to six glasses a day) and dairy intake (yogurt and cheese sticks) to her pediatrician. Soon, it was very clear that she had "developed" a horrible allergy to dairy, though it took me a long time to make the connection between her allergic symptoms—constant runny nose, nighttime cough from excessive mucous production and drainage, eczema and asthma—and her excessive dairy intake. And let's not forget the "necessary" expensive surgery to remove her adenoids and tonsils. Meanwhile, no one had yet to suggest to me that all we had to do was eliminate dairy. Did you know that human babies who drink cow milk are more likely to develop a cow milk allergy, a condition that now affects more than one in ten babies?[11]

During my third pregnancy, I actually developed a sensitivity to dairy myself. I was drinking up to three twenty-ounce glasses of milk a day and going through cheese and crackers like crazy, but thought I was doing the right thing to help my baby grow in utero. It never occurred to me that the reason I was throwing up for eight months and had impacted sinuses and horrible facial pain was all due to the inflammation and excess mucous production from overconsumption of milk.

We all need milk, right? Wrong. The dairy industry has bombarded us with propaganda for decades, leading many American parents to believe that cow milk is essential for forming healthy bones and teeth. The truth is that mammals don't need milk from any species other than their own.

We are literally brainwashed from birth that calcium from milk is essential for our kids' well-being. Yet, in actuality, milk is not a very good source of minerals. Relying solely on dairy products for calcium can lead to magnesium deficiency and other imbalances in your child's body. Milk from cows is designed to support calves, not humans.

Today, we see more and more dairy allergies, sensitivities and other chronic health issues as a result of excessive milk and formula consumption. Even though most traditionally trained ENT doctors will not directly correlate the two, I can tell you that a majority of my clients who come in with concerns about their children's health find almost immediate relief when dairy is eliminated: relief from asthma, eczema, migraines, runny nose, stomach pain, reflux, chronic cough, GERD (Gastroesophageal reflux disease) and sleep issues, to name a few. Keep in mind that if your child undergoes traditional allergy testing for milk, the test can come back negative but your child can still have what's called a "sensitivity" which can be as severe as or worse in many cases than an actual allergy. If they do have a sensitivity to milk they must be treated the same as someone with a traditional milk allergy.

The beauty of it is, no complicated, painful or expensive tests are necessary to determine if your child has an allergy or sensitivity. In addition, the long term health benefits for you and your child of not taking a daily dose of Prevacid or any other PPI (proton pump inhibitor) to help mask the symptoms of your body's reaction to dairy are well worth it. These drugs, so often prescribed for many of the symptoms listed above, can prevent your body from absorbing nutrients, potentially leading to further, more complicated health issues like possible increase risk of hip, wrist and spine fractures, anemia, low magnesium and increased risk of pneumonia (http://www.fda.gov/Drugs/Drug%20safety/InformationbyDrugClass).

As a parent, you make the choice for your child. Some kids do well on milk and I am a firm believer in all things in moderation. My middle daughter loves milk and has no adverse medical reactions, so she drinks organic milk in moderation. Pay attention to your child and their health. Are they crying a lot, constipated, not sleeping well and constantly having a runny nose?

These are all signs of either an intolerance or allergy to milk, so pull them off milk, do a test run elimination diet for several days and try a milk alternative. The results might surprise you.

DID YOU KNOW?

- As many as 50 million people in the United States are lactose intolerant including 90 percent of all Asian Americans and 75 percent of all African Americans.

- 1.3 million children in the United States have a milk allergy (this does not include all the children who suffer from milk intolerance (www.foodallergy.org)

- Until recently, the American Dairy Association and most doctors encouraged drinking four eight-ounce glasses of milk a day (I'll do the math for you: that's 1 quart of milk). They don't even tell us to eat that many vegetables, even though we probably should! Today, it's three cups, which is still 3/4 quart.

- Treating heartburn is a $10 billion dollar a year business. Why not just get off dairy?

- The federal government subsidized the milk industry to the tune of $4 billion in the past ten years (www.farm.ewg.org).

- The rate of bone fractures is highest in milk-drinking countries. Like all animal protein, milk acidifies the body pH, which triggers a biological correction causing your body to leach calcium from its own bones to bring its pH back into balance. This leaching can lead to weakened bones and possibly osteoporosis (*The New Optimum Nutrition Bible*, Patrick Holford, 1997).

Many of my clients are terrified that if they pull their kids off of milk they will become calcium deficient. Remember, dairy is not the only way to give your kids essential minerals like manganese, chromium, selenium and magnesium. You can have them snack on seeds and nuts and add crunchy vegetables like cabbage, carrots and cauliflower to their lunch boxes and dinner plates. Other great alternative sources of calcium can come from almonds, parsley, corn tortillas, prunes, pumpkin seeds, beans, bok choy, broccoli, turnip greens, mustard greens, kale and spinach.

Additional milk alternatives to cow's milk include breast milk, goat milk, organic soy milk, rice milk (my favorite and it comes in many natural flavors, like vanilla and strawberry!), hemp milk and nut milk. Just remember, babies under the age of two need to avoid nuts to possibly prevent an allergic reaction, so nut milks are not the best choice for them.

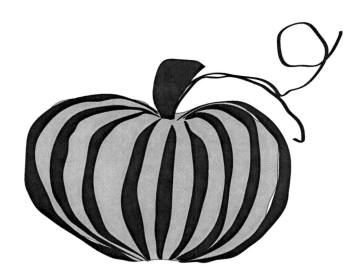

Got Beef?

As a nation, consumption of meat has increased nearly 400 percent in the past one hundred years.[12] And the average person in the United States eats over 200 pounds of meat each year.[13] This is great for the beef industry, but not so good for our kids' health. Unless you are buying organic or natural meat free from hormones, your child is consuming antibiotics, growth hormones and pesticides in every hamburger they eat, not to mention the genetically modified corn the cows are being fed.

What does this mean long-term for our children? I feel the challenge every time we eat out, as my kids love beef fajitas, hamburgers and hot dogs just like the average American child. However, according to a federal study conducted by the National Cancer Institute and Archives of Internal Medicine, heavy meat consumption increases your risk of dying from many causes, including heart disease and cancer (naturalnews.com, Monday, March 30, 2009). This scares me. Even worse, according to the People for the Ethical Treatment of Animals (PETA), feeding meat to our kids increases their chance of becoming obese and can be especially harmful to them while their bodies are still developing. The cattle our kids are eating have been fed large amount of hormones and antibiotics to make them grow faster and keep them alive in "filthy, overcrowded conditions that would otherwise kill them" (PETA). Children's bodies are especially sensitive to antibiotics and hormones and the risk to them is so great that many countries overseas have completely banned their use.

Did you know that it takes more than 2,400 gallons of water to produce one pound of meat, while growing one pound of wheat only requires twenty-five gallons? You save more water by not eating a pound of meat than you do by not showering for six months![14]

In a society surrounded by red meat everywhere we go, once again moderation is key. If you want to treat yourself to a hamburger or steak (preferably made at home and hormone-free!) go for it. Even Costco offers organic hamburgers now. But remember, with your kids it's easy to get caught in the red meat trap, especially if you eat out often as a family or tend to drive through and get fast food on the way home from work. Be aware of how much red meat your family is eating and try to keep it to a healthy level, three to four times a month at most.

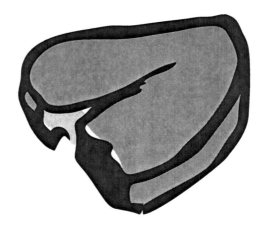

LESS MEAT: BETTER FOR YOU AND THE ENVIRONMENT

- Did you know that one ham sandwich has a carbon footprint of fourteen to thirty-four grams of CO_2?

- Eating less meat avoids polluting our streams and rivers better than any other single recycling effort.

- 70 percent of the antibiotics consumed each year in the US are given to animals on factory farms (PETA)

- An average car produces three kg/day of CO_2 and the production of one hamburger produces seventy-five kg of CO_2.[15]

- By eating less meat you help reduce the amount of methane gas produced.

- By eating less meat you also reduce the destruction of wildlife habitat, and help to save endangered species.

- Not eating meat will make you healthier. Vegetarians are less likely to get sick. They have a lower chance of getting cancer, having heart attacks and most other illnesses. They also tend to be thinner.

- Not eating meat will help to stop starvation. Meat is very energy inefficient. It takes ten times as much grain to feed a pig and then to feed a person the pig, as to simply have the person eat the grain themselves.
  (via www.kidskeeptheearthcool.org)

Government Subsidies and Food Deserts

What is a food or farm subsidy? We hear more and more today about food and farm subsidies in the media and on the internet, but many people don't fully understand what they are and how they affect us as consumers and parents. A farm subsidy is a "safety net" that the government provides to farmers to help them through the changing seasons and weather conditions to help ensure a stable food supply from year to year (EWG.org/subsidyprimer.php).

Even though the federal government claims to have these programs in place to help the farmers, most farmers do not benefit from federal farm subsidy programs, especially if their farm is a smaller one producing specialized crops. More importantly, and even more in question, is that the farmers producing fruits and vegetables are barely subsidized at all.

One of the biggest complaints nowadays is that most farm subsidies go to crops that aren't very healthy and are mostly used to produce junk food. Let's take a look at some of these crops:

1. *Corn (think HFCS)*

2. *Wheat*

3. *Soybeans*

4. *Rice*

5. *Beer*

6. *Milk*

7. *Beef*

8. *Peanut butter*

9. *Sunflower oil*

Wow! From this list, it appears that our government is subsidizing the farmers who produce all of the foods that are making us sick: HFCS from corn, gluten from wheat, soy, made from GM soybeans, potentially causing allergies. Why aren't they subsidizing the foods that we need most to be healthy? Did you know that corn subsidies in the United States totaled $77.1 billion from 1995–2010? Recent studies from various fast-food restaurants across the United States discovered that almost every cow or chicken was raised on a diet of corn, usually genetically modified corn.[16]

According to a recent PIRG study, $17 billion of the total $260 billion the government spent subsidizing agriculture went to just four common food additives: corn syrup, high fructose corn syrup, cornstarch and soy oils. Comparatively, the government spent just $261 million subsidizing apples, and far less on fruits and vegetables like spinach, broccoli and blueberries. The PIRG study explained that if the government had given taxpayers the subsidies instead of the farmers, each one would have been given $7.36 to spend on junk food and just 11 cents to spend on apples a year. This is a key factor that makes junk food more expensive than healthy food—and, by extension, that makes many Americans obese.[17]

So why is the government subsidizing what Dr. Mercola calls a "fast-food, illness-causing diet" ("The Nine Foods the Government Is Paying You to Eat," Dr. Mercola, August 3, 2011)? I ask the same question he does: Is it a coincidence that the number one source of calories in the United States, HFCS, in soda and other sugary snacks, is made from the most heavily subsidized crop—corn? Why aren't we paying the farmers to grow the foods we need to be healthy, like fruits and veggies, to make them as inexpensive and accessible as the junk food that we have access to everywhere we go? If our government is really concerned about our health as a nation and our children's health, why are they perpetuating the problem?

These are serious questions that need to be addressed sooner rather than later, before our kids get sicker and sicker.

We are beginning to hear more and more today as a nation about food deserts and what that means nutritionally for the parents and children that are forced to live and survive in them. More than 23 million Americans live at least a mile from the nearest supermarket.[18] Even when we are informed enough to make wise decisions about what to feed our family, it may still be a challenge to do so. Good food—fresh meat, dairy products and vegetables—is often not readily available and many families do not have a means of transportation to get to the neighborhoods that do offer options for purchasing healthy food. Many Americans, especially those in large urban areas, live in a "food desert," which means the closest grocery store is at least a mile away, and possibly does not have healthy choices anyway. Food deserts force people to feed their families from convenience stores and fast-food restaurants.

Government studies are starting to show that food deserts are becoming large contributors to the obesity epidemic in the United States. Those living in food deserts must walk or rely on public transportation to purchase healthy foods. But even if there was a supermarket close by, would parents choose the healthier option for their families or would they lean on fast food and convenience store items? Since there are now five fast-food restaurants for every supermarket in the United States,[19] studies are showing that even those with accessibility to large grocery stores are choosing fast food because it's easier, more convenient and addictive by design.

Think you can't afford organic food or even fruits and veggies? How much are you spending on health related medications for you or your child? Wouldn't you rather spend it on healthy food you can enjoy as a family? Don't get trapped in the cycle: you either pay for good food now or pay later with your health.

What's So Bad about the Food We Eat?

This guide is going to help you differentiate between good food and junk food. Junk food is more than the obvious offenders like candy bars, ice cream, sodas, sports drinks and fried foods. Junk food often masquerades as real food, showing up as a significant part of mealtime. Junk food is everywhere—from genetically modified seeds, to pesticide treated veggies, to meat pumped full of growth hormones. And weeding out the good from the bad can be confusing. But you're not alone. This guide will be your gateway to easy, everyday healthy eating, showing you what foods to avoid and why.

JUNK-FOOD MASQUERADERS

Junk food has made its way into every meal of the day. Learn to recognize these invaders. Some of the most common culprits include the following items:

- White Pasta
- Donuts
- Pizza
- Fish sticks
- Tater tots

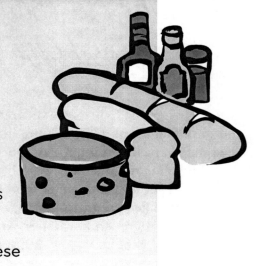

- Bologna
- Ham
- Turkey
- Hot Dogs
- Pepperoni
- Popsicles
- Sugary Cereals
- White Bread
- American cheese
- Fruit Juice
- Sports and energy drinks
- Chocolate milk
- Ketchup

Genetically Modified Foods

Genetic modification of food involves the laboratory process of artificially inserting genes into the DNA of food crops or animals. The result is called a genetically modified organism or GMO. GMOs can be engineered with genes from bacteria, viruses, insects, animals or even humans. Most Americans say that they would not eat GMOs if labeled, but unlike most other industrialized countries, the United States does not require labeling. Many people believe that the skyrocketing number of children with life-threatening allergies is associated with the introduction of GM foods into the food supply in 1990. Danger-ous soy, peanut and corn allergies have inexplicably increased exponentially in our kids over the past decade. According to Jeffrey Smith in *Seeds of Deception*, scientists believe that GM foods could lead to unexpected and hard-to-detect side effects like allergens, toxins, new diseases and nutritional problems. The FDA toxicology group wrote that GM plants could contain "un-expected high concentrations of plant toxicants." In addition, the Center for Veterinary Medicine was worried that meat and milk from animals fed GM feed (corn/soy) might be toxic.

A prime example of the danger of GM foods can be seen in soy. GM soy has been found to have seven times the amount of the known soy allergen. Next time you pick up some snack bars for your kids, or salad dressing from the store, check out the la-bels. It's hard to buy much these days that doesn't contain some derivative of soy. Most kids' snacks contain soy and several other highly allergenic ingredients like canola and cottonseed oil. My children have several friends who have life-threatening allergies to cottonseed oil and peanuts.

Although Monsanto and other big agricultural companies claim they that they are safe, the jury is definitely out on the long-term effects of GMOs and genetically engineered (GE) foods.

Did you know?

- *In thirty other countries around the world, GM foods have been banned or severely restricted?*

- *88 percent of the corn—often in the form of high fructose corn syrup—and 94 percent of the soy—think partially hydrogenated soybean oil—that we consume is genetically modified?[20]*

- *Experts estimate that more than 70 percent of processed foods in America's supermarkets contain genetically engineered ingredients.*

- *GM food is not currently tracked or labeled in our food supply so the only way to avoid it is to buy organic (see 6 Foods to Buy Organic in Section 2). It also means we can't track the long-term health implications of having it integrated into our food supply.*

FOUR TIPS FOR AVOIDING GMOS

1. Buy organic foods and produce. The produce will have a 9 as the first number in the SKU, which means it has not been genetically modified. Certified organic products cannot intentionally contain any GM ingredients.

2. Look for non-GMO project verified seals.

3. Avoid at-risk ingredients. The eight GM food crops are corn, soybeans, canola, cottonseed, sugar beets, Hawaiian papaya (most) and a small amount of zucchini and yellow squash. It may sound simple at first to avoid these foods, but when you read the labels on the processed snack bars kids like or the protein bar you prefer to eat for

breakfast, you're going to notice quite a few potentially GM ingredients. When eating out, many restaurants cook with canola oil. The alternative? Eat at home as often as possible where the food is cheaper and you know your food is clean!

4. Think about sugar. If a product is not organic and lists sugar as an ingredient, then it's usually GM coming from sugar beets and sugarcane.

5. Buy products listed on the non-GMO shopping guide at nonGMOshoppingguide. com.

Pesticides and Herbicides

As parents, it's important to be aware of how our food is grown. We are what we eat and, currently, there are over 3,500 man-made chemicals in our food supply.

Most food that is grown in the United States—organic is the exception—has been depleted of nutrients by herbicides, pesticides and sewage sludge.

These herbicides and pesticides are also called "anti-nutrients" by the medical profession as they keep our bodies from absorbing and using the nutrients from the food we eat. Some feel that these anti-nutrients play a key role in many of today's diseases.

What Every Mom Should Know about Pesticides

- Pesticides are invisible, odorless, and tasteless, so the only way to know that a food is pesticide free is to buy organic. Even then, you should use a vegetable and fruit wash before eating produce. I like Veggie Wash (www.veggie-wash.com) which uses natural organic citrus solvents to clean fruit and vegetables. You can also make your own with vinegar and salt.

- Organic foods have a higher nutritional value: an organic apple has as much as 300 percent more vitamin C and 60 percent greater calcium content than a conventional apple. Buy them in season and organic produce is very affordable.

- Pesticide exposure is linked to memory decline, Parkinson's disease and depression, among other illnesses.

- Pesticides cross the placenta and go to the fetus.

- 800 to 1000 farmers and farm workers die every year from exposure to pesticides.[21]

- *Pesticides are toxic to both human beings and the environment.*

- *Women with high levels of the common pesticide DDT in their blood are four times as likely to develop breast cancer as women with low levels.[22]*

- *Pesticides are known to harm the nervous and endocrine systems as well as deplete the Earth's protective ozone layer, which can lead to skin cancer. They are carcinogenic as well.*

- *The EPA says pesticides block the body's uptake of nutrients critical for proper growth and wreak havoc on development by permanently altering the way a child's system functions.*

- *Understand the vocabulary: "Conventional" means pesticides were used. "Organic" means 95 percent of the product contains no pesticides. 100 percent organic means the product contains no pesticides at all.*

- *In addition to common fruits and vegetables, teas, potatoes, tomatoes, peanuts and coffee are also highly treated with pesticides.*

- *Try to go organic the first trimester of your pregnancy: studies now show that pesticides/ herbicides are linked to autism and gestational diabetes.[23]*

A Gallon of Chemicals a Year

From *The UltraMind Solution*, by Dr. Mark Hyman:

> *The average American consumes a gallon of neu-rotoxic pesticides and herbicides each year by eating conventionally grown fruits and vegetables. One study showed children who regularly ate nonorganic foods purchased in an average grocery store had high levels of pesticides in their urine, while those who ate strictly organic food had almost none. Other studies link early pesticide exposure to autism and other neurobehavioral problems in children.*

The toxins used to make processed food last on the shelf for years contribute to weight gain, obesity, diabetes and reduced metabolism. Our body doesn't recognize these chemicals as real food, so it holds onto them and stores them in the fatty tissue of our bodies. This is called bioaccumulation and can eventually make us sick.

Unfortunately, it doesn't look like pesticides are going away anytime soon. But as parents, we can keep our kids free of pesticides by becoming aware of the foods we buy. Each time you choose organic produce or other natural products, you are casting a vote with your dollars, sending a message demanding cleaner foods. And as the demand for organic and natural food increases, the costs will decrease, making it more affordable for everyone.

Why Raising Our Kids with Healthy Eating Habits Is So Challenging in the United States

One of the things that disturbs me the most as a mom and nutritional consultant is that on the outside, the food industry appears to be advocating for our health—"Milk, it does a body good!"—while behind the scenes, something dramatically different is happening. It would seem that the great lure for profitability and the American dollar has overcome the conscience of most companies in the food industry. Simultaneously, the media perpetuates these myths by creating ad campaigns targeted toward children that position unhealthy foods as healthy options.

Children under the age of ten believe what they see and hear as the truth exactly as it is presented to them, unless told otherwise by a respected adult. Example: buy frosted flakes, "They're GRRREEEAT!" As a result, American children are gaining weight at an alarming rate and developing early signs of diabetes, high blood pressure and heart disease as well as many other behavioral disorders at an extremely young age.

Marketing to kids and parents is big business. These companies are counting on what author Marion Nestle calls the "pester factor." In her book *What to Eat*, she describes this as persistent nagging from kids that's guaranteed to wear parents down. Marketing campaigns give kids the idea that they are supposed to eat packaged foods rather than unprocessed home-cooked foods because it's more fun—think Lunchables. They also want kids to expect foods to be sweet and salty and to come in fun colors, shapes and packages. This excess consumption of sweet and salty foods distorts our kids' taste buds and makes our lives as parents much more challenging, especially when we are simply trying to get our kids to eat a fresh piece of broccoli.

We see pictures of happy modern families eating fast food everywhere we look. Is fast food the new "normal" in your family?

When my first daughter was born and I needed a few moments to myself to take a shower or fold laundry, I would let her watch Baby Einstein or some other short educational video, but never any commercials. As time went by and more children seemed to appear out of nowhere at our house, I found myself slipping and letting them watch more TV, which led to the dreaded commercials. I was now faced with what every mother in America has to deal with: a small child telling me why a certain toy or food was essential to her happiness. I also noticed that the more TV they watched, the worse their behavior became as they spent less time outside getting energy out and using their brains to look for doodle bugs and play "spies" in the backyard. I began to find myself negotiating with said small child more often than I cared to, which was when I put two and two together, and everything came to a screeching halt.

That began what I lovingly refer to as the "Dark Ages" in our home. No screens during the week. Period. At that point, they

"You are what you eat, drink and think...so what does that make you?"

—GABRIELLE WELCH

were young enough, one, three and four, that no one had any school-related projects to do on the computer, so a screen-free home was possible.

The first week was brutal but once they understood that the TV was "closed" during the week, they bought it. It has worked well for years and we still adhere to it today with a seven, nine and eleven-year-old. Without a TV, my kids were not only free from the brainwashing that happens on the shows themselves, but they were also kept at a distance from all the commercials for sugary cereals and junky snacks, which made food shopping so much nicer. They didn't request those items because they had no idea they existed. The same rule goes for fast food. They have no clue what it is until someone introduces it to them. If you make it clear to family and friends that the drive-thru is not an option for your child, you will be shocked at how long your little ones can live without knowing what it is. Or, you may choose to take matters into your own hands and share your thoughts on fast food with your children every time you pass a fast-food restaurant.

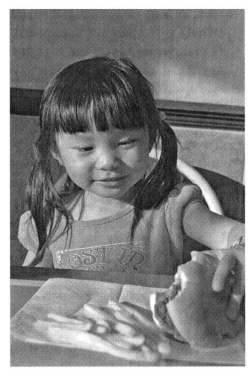

My clients, as well as most of my friends with young children, face the same issues. It's nearly impossible to walk through a store without being badgered by your child who has seen thousands of commercials over the past week—unless you invoke the Welch rule of no screens during the week.

Comparison to European Nations

In the United States, food companies can add preservatives, dyes and other harmful ingredients to their products, while many other countries in Europe have banned the use of such toxins. For example, the Kraft Lunchables that you buy in the United States is loaded with nitrates (preservatives), food coloring and MSG while kids overseas are getting a chemical-free, hormone-free, antibiotic-free lunch with real cheese and real ham. How does this happen?

Most of the countries in Europe, as well as many in Africa, New Zealand and Australia have banned the importing of US foods that have been genetically modified or contain food coloring and artificial additives and preservatives. When food coloring is used, European products are required to use warning labels that say "consumption may have an adverse effect on activity and attention in children." Don't we want that here in the US for OUR children?

That's right: parents and government officials in other countries made their voices heard, put their foot down and insisted that large companies like Kraft, Wal-Mart and Coke remove these harmful chemicals from their products before they would allow them to be sold in their respective countries.

Many parents and health experts here in our country have understood the effects of artificial colors for years, but the US Food and Drug Administration has not acknowledged these adverse health effects. Currently, US companies add artificial colors to everyday foods and products like children's and adult medications, hot dogs and even cereal just to make them an attractive color so kids will beg their parents to buy them. But think about it, for a child who is allergic to red food dye, what could be worse than giving him allergy or other medication that's red when he is sick? It doesn't make any sense.

In an already crazy-busy world, wouldn't it make our lives much easier as parents to not have to worry about every morsel of food our kids are putting into their bodies? We need to become parent activists, making our mark in any way that we can, in our homes and even on a local, statewide or national level.

Family Challenges

As parents, we juggle a lot—making sure that homework is finished, chores are done, tummies are fed and bodies are washed. We can end up feeling guilty because we had to rush to accomplish everything on our list.

Often we can't even be patient with our spouse—or ourselves—because we have been assaulted by our kids' needs all day. We have nothing left to give. We are an empty vending machine. Yet now we have to face the dishes, the laundry, cleaning the bathroom and taking care of the pets. This stress permeates our lives.

Stress has an incredible impact on our energy and on how and what decisions we make. Stress can make you want to grab a breakfast taco or donut for your kids instead of making breakfast. Or it can make you want to skip breakfast completely and just throw the kids some money to grab something out of the vending machine. If you are stressed your kids will feel it. Children are very intuitive and pick up on our emotions. In Section 3, I offer ideas and suggestions to reduce stress in your home so that neither you nor your child is sucked into the trap of emotional eating.

No Time for Dinner

In the past fifteen years, we have trended dramatically toward fewer organized meals at home, more fast food and soft drinks, larger portion sizes and more snacking because food is everywhere. These eating habits promote higher calorie intake from less nutritious foods.

What are some of the reasons why we don't have time to make a family dinner and share a meal with our kids?

- *We are constantly getting home late from work and our kids' sports events.*

- *We don't like to cook and we get frazzled making even the simplest things.*

- *We get overwhelmed when we have to grocery shop, especially when there are kids involved.*

- *We forget to go to the store and can't handle the thought of going with all the kids at five o'clock.*

- *We are managing several kids on different schedules.*

Everything seems to happen at the last minute. We often feel like we don't have time for anything. This is because we have too much on our plates and refuse to say no, to the point of exhaustion.

We are wiped out again and our spouse is working late, so why bother cooking? Just order a pizza. It's easy and the kids will be happy.

It is important to determine how stress affects your family, especially around mealtime. We need to understand how time—or lack of it—affects us as individuals and as families. Feeling stressed and anxious leads to more mealtime battles, more arguing, less patience, less focus and less concentration on homework and class work. And giving in to highly processed TV dinners and take-out food leads to weight and health issues.

The Time Is Now

We have allowed convenience to take the place of real food. As parents, sometimes convenience can be a lifesaver, but how far are we willing to go? More often than not, convenience foods are the worst for us: processed, prepackaged foods devoid of any nutrients. We live in a nation of overfed and undernourished kids: overfed because there is no sense of proper portions anymore so our children eat way more than their size can allow, and undernourished because the nutritional value of the foods they are eating is nonexistent. If we don't do our part to make a change we will all be facing serious consequences sooner rather than later.

It is our responsibility to talk to our kids about food and making good choices as much as the media does. Are we talking to them as much about the dangers of processed junk food as we are about sex, drugs and alcohol?

If we don't make some drastic changes in the way that we are feeding our children, we are going to be spending more and more money on doctor visits and drugs for problems that can be eradicated simply by eating clean and real food.

Now you know the State of the Nation. It's time to learn what you can do to change it, one household at a time, starting with your own.

In the next two sections, I will provide you with critical information and guidelines on what foods to avoid when you are shopping and why. I'll also give you the inside scoop on how to spot tricksters, swindlers and fakers: three terms I've created to help you better understand the harmful additives that are in much of the food your kids eat and how to easily avoid them.

In Section 2, we'll visit the infamous "Kids' Menu" and learn what lurks in the food our kids are offered whenever we eat out. I'll give you better alternatives and show you that it's possible to eat out and eat healthy.

Finally, in Section 3, we'll look at the importance of buying organic, seasonal foods, as well as behavior modification tips that will help you end mealtime battles.

With the information provided in this guide, you'll be able to get your family on the road to health in no time.

Let's get started!

"Bad diet is to the US what lead pipes were to the Romans —a hidden killer."

—EMERSON HANKAMER

What's Really in Our Food and How to Keep Your Kids Safe

When it comes to guiding their children along a path of healthy eating, American parents face a remarkable challenge. From genetically modified foods, to artificial sugars, to toxic additives like MSG and food coloring and cheap substitutes like high fructose corn syrup, our kids are consuming harmful ingredients at practically every meal. Most parents don't recognize the effects of toxic eating until it is too late—until their children are sick or allergic or undernourished. Fake foods—foods made with unnatural, processed ingredients—have become the new normal. They're seen on kids' menus, in school cafeterias and at ballpark and movie concession stands.

But there is hope. You can change the way your kids eat. In this section, I will help you to understand why these everyday foods are so dangerous and give you easy-to-use tips for substituting nutritious, whole foods for the worst offenders. As a mother, you have the ability to guide your kids to a lifetime of healthy eating. By educating ourselves—and our families—about what's really in the food our kids are eating and creating a dining plan that works for everyone, our children will regularly be consuming foods that will help them reach their fullest potential.

It's easier than you think! I will provide you with quick and easy tools for everyday eating, outlining foods to avoid and foods to buy—including when to buy them and why they are beneficial for your children.

Be a Food Sleuth

Big food companies are really sneaky these days, since they know that many moms are determined to avoid junk food. That's why it's more important than ever to be armed with the knowledge and tools necessary to be a food sleuth. It's impossible to crack the food code unless you know what you're looking for. I'll help you identify what to detect on food labels (and tell you how to teach your kids as well!) so you can learn to avoid the manipulation of major food companies.

Understanding what foods you can trust, like packaged food with fewer than five ingredients, or produce with the number 9 at the beginning of the SKU to indicate organic is key. But the most efficient way of ensuring that your family consumes only wholesome, healthy foods is to read food labels like an expert. "Who has the time to stand in the grocery aisle and read each label?" you ask. If you care about your family's health—you will find the time. Understanding food labels is the only way to distinguish junk food from the real thing. That can be tough to do in a day and age where no one *wants* you to understand what's on the label. To help you determine what foods to avoid when grocery shopping for the week or eating on the go, I've compiled a list of the most common *tricksters, swindlers* and *fakers*—harmful additives and chemicals that make their way into the foods your kids eat. Once you learn what they are and where they're found, you can teach your family how to steer clear of dangerous ingredients.

FACT:
Did you know that obese children are two times more likely to die before the age of 55?

Tricksters

Tricksters are additives, food substitutes or chemicals that trick the body into wanting more food, our brain cells into becoming overexcited, or our hormones into doing something they wouldn't normally do. Over time, these chemically induced reactions can kill brain cells, cause cancer, Alzheimer's, diabetes, seizures, heart palpitations, anxiety, obesity and osteoporosis, among other illnesses.[1]

Let's look at the three main tricksters—aspartame, MSG and parabens—and learn how to keep them out of our kids' diets.

Aspartame

Aspartame is an artificial sweetener usually found in food like kids' yogurt, breakfast cereals, sugar-free gum, some desserts and most diet drinks and is sadly a significant part of the Standard American Diet. Since most Americans consume at least two hundred calories a day from soda (http://www.cdc.gov/nchs/data/databriefs/db71.htm), one of the first things most Americans do when they want to lose weight is switch from regular soda to diet soda. Unfortunately, this creates the opposite effect and most people, including our kids, end up gaining, not losing weight. Here is a basic run down: aspartame is made of aspartic acid (40%), phenylalanine (50%) and methanol (10%). Without getting too technical, aspartate is a neurotransmitter and when we have too much of it, it becomes an excitotoxin, which means it excites brain cells to death. When we lose more than 75 percent of our brain cells in certain parts of the brain, we start seeing symptoms of chronic illness. In addition to the diseases and conditions mentioned above, aspartame has also been connected to multiple sclerosis, dementia and ALS (Lou Gehrig's disease). Children and pregnant women are especially susceptible to excitotoxins.[2]

Studies show that people who drink aspartame have higher than normal levels of phenylalanine, which is an amino acid found in our brain. High levels of phenylalanine lowers serotonin production, which can lead to depression. Did you know that one in ten Americans take an antidepressant? [3] Do you want your child to be one of those people?

> Moms, more and more of our children are becoming depressed. We are currently facing a crisis where American kids are becoming "overfat, underfit and unhappy" (for more on this, read **Dr. Sears' LEAN Kids**: these are the terms he uses to describe kids today). When kids are overfat from ingesting too many chemicals that upset the delicate hormonal balance in their bodies—like aspartame—they become unhappy and stressed. Stress promotes fat storage, increased chance of illness, negatively affects sleep and can lead to depression.[4] Be part of the solution, not part of the problem and keep chemicals like aspartame away from your kids so they can enjoy the happy, healthy childhood they deserve.

Aspartame: What You Need to Know

Artificial sweeteners like NutraSweet and Equal have been a topic of controversy since they hit the supermarket shelves over thirty years ago. There were those who were excited to have a healthy sugar substitute and those who were immediately skeptical as to its safety. Who wouldn't want a healthy sugar alternative? The key word is healthy.

Artificial sweeteners trick the tongue into thinking it's tasting something sweet. Did you know that aspartame is 200 times sweeter per molecule than sugar?

Unfortunately, our bodies are smarter than we are. If we try to fill a sweet craving with "fake" sugar instead of an apple for instance, we might feel briefly satisfied, but as soon as our body figures out we didn't give it what it wanted, the cravings return and we reach for another diet soda, starting the process all over again.

Although we all thought that we were off the hook by switching to a diet soda, little did we know that aspartame contributes to weight *gain* by stimulating the appetite and creating a craving for carbohydrates, especially the kind high in fat and processed sugar—like the donut and the bagel. The American Cancer Society says that people who use artificial sweeteners gain more weight than those who don't drink them![5]

In addition, aspartame contains methanol, which the body breaks down into formaldehyde when it reaches eighty-six degrees. Since our average body temperature is 98.6, this process

> **FACT:**
> Did you know the brain is the most food sensitive organ in the body?

occurs every time you consume it. When you consume aspartame, you are slowly embalming yourself over time as the sugar substitute increases formaldehyde buildup in cells—the fancy word for this process is bioaccumulation.

Moms, think twice next time you offer your child a diet drink! You may think you're doing them a favor by cutting the calories, but there is a larger price to pay. According to recent research, aspartame may account for up to 75 percent of dangerous food reactions reported to the FDA.

Aspartame: Where It Lurks

Many foods labeled "sugar-free" contain aspartame. Most of them are foods your kids like, which can make them more difficult to avoid, but definitely not impossible.

Here is a short list of some of the most common offenders:

- *Sugar-free gelatin*

- *Breakfast cereal*

- *Diet drinks*

- *Sugar-free candy*

- *Sugar-free desserts like pudding*

- *Sugar-free gum*

- *Hot chocolate mix*

- *Breath mints*

- *Sweetened teas*

- *Yogurt*

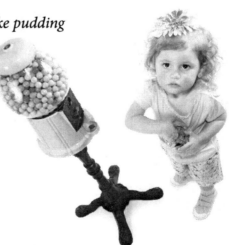

DIET DRINKS

Diet drinks not only contain aspartame, but also leach calcium from bones and can be a huge contributor to osteoporosis. Have you noticed how your friend who sips diet drinks all day—instead of eating—looks hunched over at a very early age? Diet drinks also contain a high amount of phosphorus. According to Michael Murray, ND, higher levels of phosphorus can lower the calcium in your body and this can prevent absorption of the amount needed for bones to remain strong. Dr. Murray points out that this leads to poor bone mineralization in children and a higher risk of osteoporosis in adults.[6] Keep your kids away from anything sugar-free as often as you can. If you want a tasty soda substitute, combine three-quarters sparkling water with a quarter cranberry juice. It's healthy and tastes great! Visit www.sodastreamusa.com to learn how to save money and make your own soda at home.

MSG

(Monosodium Glutamate, aka "natural flavors," hydrolyzed protein, autolyzed yeast and many other sneaky names).

OTHER SNEAKY WORDS FOR MSG

(or items that contain it):

- *Glutamate*
- *Textured protein*
- *Monosodium glutamate*
- *Hydrolyzed protein*
- *Monopotassium glutamate (any protein that is hydrolyzed)*
- *Glutamic acid*
- *Yeast extract*
- *Calcium caseinate*
- *Yeast food*
- *Sodium caseinate*
- *Autolyzed yeast*
- *Gelatin*
- *Yeast nutrient*

(www.truthinlabeling.org)

MSG is also a common *trickster*. It tricks your nervous system into thinking the foods you are eating are tastier than they really are, so you eat more (think: "No one can eat just one."). Aside from tricking your body into wanting more than it needs, MSG (like aspartame) is also an excitotoxin that can damage children's brains by killing brain cells and affecting the development of the nervous system so that years later they may have learning and emotional difficulties—ADD, ADHD or autism—or hormonal problems. Everyone has a different tolerance level for these chemical substitutes or additives, so you might not know

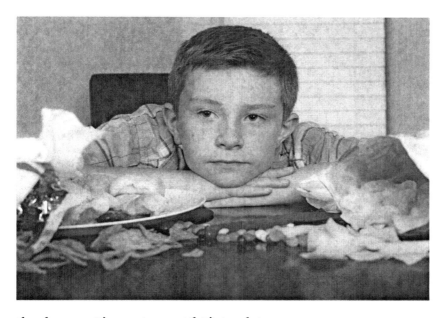

the damage it's causing until it's too late. Like aspartame, cumulative exposure to MSG can lead to neurodegenerative disorders like Alzheimer's, Parkinson's, ALS and Huntington's disease. A medical study done at Washington University School of Medicine by Dr. John Olney, a leading researcher in the field, determined that "the MSG in a single bowl of commercial soup consumed with a can of diet soda, which contains aspartame, would raise a two-year-old's blood level of MSG to six times the concentration demonstrated to cause brain damage in animals."[7] I don't know about you, but that's enough to make me steer clear of MSG and avoid giving it to my kids whenever possible.

Behaviors associated with artificial colors are mood swings, hyperactivity, problems concentrating, and the inability to control their emotions.

MSG SAVVY

MSG is rarely labeled as such on food labels anymore. The big food companies are smarter than that. They have created other misleading terminology for MSG, words like "natural flavors," "maltodextrin" or "hydrolyzed yeast protein." "Food manufacturers are not stupid. They've caught on to the fact that people like you want to avoid eating this nasty food additive. As a result, do you think they responded by removing MSG from their products? Well, a few may have, but most of them just tried to 'clean' their labels. In other words, they tried to hide the fact that MSG is an ingredient."[8]

Real food never contains MSG. Have you ever heard of an apple or a piece of broccoli enhanced with MSG? Of course not! That's because they don't *need* to be enhanced to taste good. Fruits and veggies taste good by design.

MSG is often found in these common food items:

- *Canned soups*

- *Snack chips*

- *Bottled salad dressing*

- *Instant noodle soups*

- *Sports drinks*

- *Soy sauce*

- *Hot dogs*

- *Snack bars and protein bars*

- *Candy*

- *Seasoning salt*

- *Many spice mixes*

Truthfully, I have been hard pressed lately to find much that doesn't have MSG. The kids and I are constantly surprised to find MSG in food and drinks that are advertised as "natural" or healthy. Most recently, we were on a summer road trip and my ten-year-old daughter picked up a fruit and nut bar I had bought at a local health food store to snack on during our trip. I had skimmed the label, which had very few ingredients, and thought it looked clean. But no! She pointed out that it had "natural flavors." Is one time an issue? No. One snack bar is not the problem. But recurring use over many years can lead to serious health problems down the road.

That means as moms, we have to be even more diligent in being sleuths and giving our kids clean, unprocessed, unpackaged food.

GOMASIO SEAWEED SALT

Organic Gomasio Seaweed Salt by Eden Foods is one of the secret weapons in my pantry. Most Americans are unaware of the importance of sea vegetables in our diet, and the SAD diet most of our kids are on **definitely** does not include them. At a time with kids' sodium levels rapidly on the rise, seaweed salt is a great alternative for seasoning your kids' food that won't lead to hypertension.

Organic Gomasio Seaweed Salt and other Gomasio condiments (edenfoods.com) are a great way to get these into your kids diets. Whether you use them on a stir fry, salads, in soups or as a seasoning for chicken, pork or beef, it's an easy and tasty way to incorporate these essential vitamins and minerals into your kids' diets. Also for moms, in an age where more and more of us are suffering from low thyroid problems due to lack of iodine, Gomasio may help regulate your thyroid as well.

Besides iodine, sea vegetables are rich sources of iron, magnesium, potassium, boron, silica, selenium and chromium. They are also loaded with essential fatty acids, vitamins (including vitamin D) and water soluble fibers which make them excellent bone-building and tissue repairing foods.

Finally, sea vegetables have a *powerful detoxifying effect* on the body; not only do they absorb toxins and heavy metals, they also reduce inflammation. The best news is, it tastes great and can be found on the salt aisle in your local grocery store.

Parabens

Parabens are preservatives used in personal care products as well as in food items—this is particularly scary. What? You want to know how we could possibly be eating something that we also may be rubbing into our skin or using to wash our hair?

Well, it's true. Parabens are used in both food and many other items we use in our daily personal care regimen. Here's the problem: our skin is porous. When we absorb parabens into the body through the skin, they act as endocrine disruptors, which means they mimic our hormones while at the same time *tricking* our actual hormones so they don't know what to do anymore. The result? Hormone imbalance! Note: Hormones are very important to our bodies. Not only do they play a major role in fertility, but they also affect our ability to sleep, how we manage stress and many other critical brain and bodily functions.[9] Remember, 90 percent of a child's brain development happens between the ages of birth to five years. When children's hormones are disrupted by parabens, it can dramatically alter their sleep, behavior, mood and ability to learn at a critical time in their brain development.

It's important to know that parabens are now also directly linked to cancer. Parabens can mimic the hormone estrogen, which is known to play a role in the development of breast cancers. In addition, a medical study published in the July 2012 issue of the *Journal of Applied Technology* shows even more of a correlation between parabens and breast cancer.

The study was entitled "Measurement of paraben concentrations in human breast tissue at serial locations across the breast from axilla to sternum," and was led by Dr. Philippa Darbre from the University of Reading in the UK. The study found that virtually all—99 percent—of the tissue samples collected from women participating in the study contained at least one paraben, and 60 percent of the samples contained no less than five parabens.[10]

Parabens are usually found in personal care products like shampoos and soaps, but can also be found in the following common foods:

- *Jelly*

- *Soft drinks*

- *Beer*

- *Cake*

- *Salad dressings*

- *Cereal or potato-based snacks*

- *Coated nuts*

- *Liquid dietary food supplements*

When shopping for personal care items, read your labels. It's now quite easy to find shampoos and soaps that are paraben-free at a very reasonable price. Whole Foods 365 brand has a great line of soaps, conditioners and shampoos that are affordable *and* paraben-free and even big names like Johnson & Johnson are now offering healthier personal care products for babies and children as well. To research the products you are currently using on your kids for their safety level or to seek out the safety of new products, check out Environmental Working Group's cosmetic database at: www.ewg.org/skindeep/.

Swindlers

Swindlers are cheap ingredients that big food companies use to save money. They make processed food products extra tasty by also adding *tricksters* like MSG so our bodies get hooked and we keep going back for more. A good example of this is the genetically modified soy they use to fill hamburgers or the thirty-eight ingredients they use to make a chicken nugget. Yes, thirty-eight—one of which is an "antifoaming agent" which is also used in shampoos. That's just gross.

Let's take a look at some of the more common *swindlers* and how to avoid them.

Partially Hydrogenated Oils
(Trans fats)

Did you know that 40 percent of the products found in a typical US supermarket contain trans fat? Not only do you have to worry about your kids ingesting it if you decide to make a quick last-minute dash through the drive-thru, you have to be on the lookout for it at the grocery store as well.

Partially hydrogenated oils or trans fats are rarely found in nature but occur often in the production of processed food in the United States. We hear about the danger of them constantly now and have to be on the lookout when we are shopping for our families.

Consuming partially hydrogenated oils is like in-haling cigarette smoke. They will kill you—slowly, over time, but as surely as you breathe. And in the mean-time, they will make you fat! Unlike butter or virgin co-conut oil, hydrogenated oils contain high levels of trans fats. A trans fat is an otherwise normal fatty acid that has been "transmogrified" by high-heat processing of a free oil. In short, trans fats are poisons, just like arsenic or cyanide. They interfere with the metabolic processes of life by taking the place of a natural substance that performs a critical function. And that is the definition of a poison. Your body has no defense against them, because they never even existed in our two billion years of evolution—so we've never had the need or the oppor-tunity to evolve a defense against them.

—Eric Armstrong at Treelight.com

Trans fats are also *tricksters* because they trick your body into eating more food in hopes of getting the essential fatty acids it needs. If you are consuming lots of saturated fats on a daily basis, like French fries, burgers, too much cheese or processed meats, there is a very strong chance that you or your children will become overweight and eventually sick. To stay healthy and keep our bodies at an ideal weight, we need to eat foods with large amounts of **polyunsaturated** oils—which contain essential fatty acids—like fish, olives, nuts and egg yolks. In addition, we should supplement our diet with an over-the-counter fish or krill oil, like those made by Nordic Naturals (nordicnaturals.com) or BodyBioBalance, a plant based oil, (bodybio.com). Unlike trans fats, over time, these healthy foods with polyunsaturated fats actually decrease your sense of hunger.

Our bodies don't make all the essential fatty acids we need. As a result, we need to get some of them from our food and through supplementation. Did you know that in addition to giving our kids a 500-1000 mg fish oil supplement every day, it's still recommended that they consume up to twelve ounces of wild caught fish once a week to get the right amount of EFA's for their growing brains? My kids take fish oil pills every day or the liquid oil in a smoothie and we work each week to get those twelve ounces of fish into their diet.

In addition, partially hydrogenated oils cause weight gain the same way that saturated fats do—they trick your body, by making you consume even more fat to get the essential fatty acids you need. But partially hydrogenated fats are even worse: they are also "blockers." Not only do they make you sick over time by raising your "bad" cholesterol and lowering your "good" cholesterol, they also interfere with the body's ability to ingest and utilize the good fats!

GET SAVVY ABOUT SOYBEAN OIL

Most partially hydrogenated oil is partially hydrogenated *soybean* oil, which is often also genetically modified. Soybean oil depresses the thyroid—and when your thyroid is low, your energy level is low, you feel less like exercising and you can gain weight more easily. Partially hydrogenated oil is in almost everything because it's cheaper than butter and the government still allows it to be put into our food in mass quantities. When you eat out, restaurant breads and fried foods are also loaded with it. Because of the prevalence of some derivatives of soybean oil, especially in kids' snacks, our kids are consuming soybean oil—partially *hydrogenated* soybean oil—in virtually everything they eat. Coincidentally, as a nation we are experiencing epidemic levels of diabetes, obesity, heart disease, and cancer not only in adults but in children as well.[11]

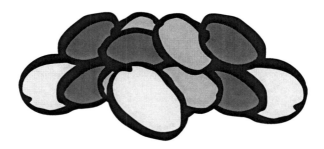

Trans fats are dangerous, and are what you usually get if you opt for fast food—except at Chick-fil-A because they have opted for a healthier peanut oil. Trans fats raise our bad cholesterol and lower our good cholesterol and because they can damage cells and cause inflammation, they can lead to cancer, arthritis and many other chronic illnesses.[12]

Partially hydrogenated soybean oil, in particular, can lead to serious lifelong allergies in kids and many other chronic illnesses. The majority of the soy in the United States is genetically modified and we still have no long-term studies telling us what damage it's doing to our kids and us. The short-term studies tell us that it's one of the leading causes of the exponential increase in asthma, autism, ADHD and allergies in kids over the past decade.[13]

Partially hydrogenated oils are often found in these common food items:

- *Supermarket muffins*
- *Donuts*
- *Bread*
- *Margarine*
- *Vegetable shortening*
- *Ice cream*
- *Ready-made pies*
- *Biscuits and crackers*
- *Cakes*
- *Cake mixes*
- *Tortillas*
- *Pizza (One more way to fall into the Pizza Trap!)*
- *Mayonnaise*
- *Salad dressings*
- *Chips*
- *Artificial creamer (Avoid this like the plague as it's full of tricksters, swindlers and fakers . . . just stick with good old fashioned organic half-and-half.)*

GHEE IS BETTER BUTTER

Ghee is considered to be the very best fat one can eat. It is made up of short chain fatty acids and is easily assimilated, even helping in the digestion and assimilation of other foods. Ghee has one of the highest 'flash points' of any oil (485 deg) and is exquisite for sautéing. Before the advent of commercial vegetable oils, ghee was widely used for deep frying. Unlike other butter-based products, ghee has a high smoking point and can be stored without refrigeration for weeks. Ghee is shelf stable and is only affected by sunlight and/or water. Ghee is known to increase intelligence, refine the intellect and improve the memory (Adapted from *"Ghee is life"—Sarva Darsana Sangraha*).

Ghee (rhymes with key), also known as clarified butter, can be bought premade at the grocery store and can also be easily made at home. Simply melt four sticks of organic unsalted butter in a pan, then leave on medium heat for thirty minutes. It should bubble and pop, but not turn brown. You can watch the white solids come to the top. After thirty minutes, remove from the heat and let it sit for a few minutes, then strain into a glass jar. The good news is, this process also removes all the lactose from the butter. So those of you who are lactose-intolerant or have lactose intolerant kids should be able to enjoy the ghee with no negative side effects.

71

High Fructose Corn Syrup

High fructose corn syrup (HFCS), by definition, is a "potent form of sugar that is sweeter than regular sugar, increases appetite, promotes obesity more than regular sugar and is more addictive than cocaine."[14]

The ratio of fructose (55 percent) to glucose (45 percent) wreaks havoc on our bodies and differentiates HFCS from plain sugar. Fructose is a carbohydrate, but metabolizes like a fat. It's a toxin and is metabolized by the liver, not the brain, which can lead to serious health issues, starting with obesity.[15]

Ghrelin is the hunger hormone that sends a signal to your brain when you are full, to tell your body to quit eating. This hormone is suppressed when you eat something with HFCS because of the altered ratios of fructose to glucose. So what happens when your kids are eating junk food and soda full of HFCS while parked in front of the TV? It's a biochemical reaction! They never feel full, and they aren't being mindful, so they keep eating. Did you know that the earlier you expose kids to refined sugar, or HFCS, the more they will crave it later?

Fructose is a chronic hepatotoxin, which is a fancy way of saying it's like alcohol without the buzz.[16] HFCS can also increase the blood level of triglycerides, the fats that clog arteries and contribute to cardiovascular disease. The United States is the highest consumer of HFCS in the world and we are also ranked toward the top in obesity, type II diabetes and cardiovascular disease.[17] See any correlation?

High fructose corn syrup is also found in some baby formulas. This may explain the recent epidemic of obese six month olds. If the HFCS suppresses ghrelin, the enzyme that helps them to realize they are full, what's to stop a baby from consuming formula until they projectile vomit because they've eaten too much?

Research shows that when babies aren't allowed to establish their own hunger and feeding cues from birth, they will likely struggle with overeating for the rest of their lives.[18] HFCS corn syrup is sweeter and cheaper to produce than cane syrup so it's an easy choice for the mass production of baby formula until we step up and do something about it. However, the good news is that HFCS is usually only found in lactose free and soy based formulas.

Most doctors and nutritionists agree that the number one cause of the childhood obesity epidemic is the prevalence and over consumption of HFCS in soft drinks and sports or energy drinks. This goes back to the biochemical reaction to HFCS versus the natural sugars found in fruits, vegetables or milk-based formulas.[19]

COCONUT WATER: NATURE'S SPORTS DRINK

One summer day at the pool, my friend Margie and I were lamenting the beverage choices geared toward kids. We wondered how we were going to get through the season with kids begging and whining for sports drinks and juice. She said, "What about coconut water, nature's sports drink?" I had definitely known about and tried coconut water, but never really thought of offering it to my kids, even though many brands come in individual size boxes with straws. So I decided to do some research.

Coconut water has been used for centuries in tropical areas for hydration. It is naturally sweet and low in calories. It is rich in electrolytes, which is why many people today use it before, during, or after a workout. It also has fifteen times the potassium of a banana. Coconut water was even used as an IV during WWII and the Vietnam War to rehydrate our soldiers when supplies were low. The electrolyte levels of coconut water are very similar to human blood, so it was safe for doctors to insert it directly into their blood stream. WOW! And to think that our kids are being taught that chocolate milk is the best way to rehydrate after being on the playground for thirty minutes—sad but true.

When you give thirsty kids coconut water, you aren't pumping them full of sugars, food dye or excess sodium. The best news is—it tastes great. We like ZICO's all-natural coconut water, Amy and Brian Coconut Juice with Pulp and the highly rated Harmless Harvest 100% Organic Raw Coconut Water.

HOMEMADE SODA

As an alternative to store-bought sodas or sports drinks loaded with HFCS, try mixing pure juices with sparkling water, or dilute a sports drink with 1/3 sparkling water or club soda. My kids love having a glass with 1/3 Simply Lemonade and 2/3 club soda at home, or when we go out to eat, they'll have one part cranberry juice and two parts club soda. This also works really well as a sports drink alternative (no MSG, food dye or aspartame!) when your kids have been out on the field for an hour and want something cold and sweet. If they don't like bubbles, just use water.

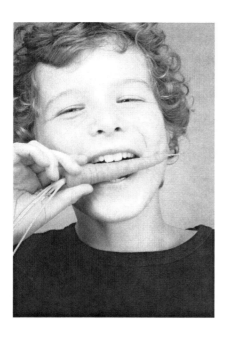

FACT: Did you know there is more sugar in an 8 oz carton of chocolate milk than in a can of soda?

According to recent statistics, eighty-six percent of corn produced in the United States is genetically modified. Although the corn industry states otherwise, many nutrition experts and food activists feel that GM corn turned into HFCS is still genetically modified and therefore harmful. HFCS is the go-to now for large snack and soft drink companies because HFCS is very cheap for companies to use since corn in the United States is highly subsidized.[20] That means *we* are paying for it. I don't know about you, but I personally don't want to pay for something that I don't even want my kids eating! For years the federal government has subsidized corn, costing billions of dollars a year. Much of America's heartland is covered by endless rows of corn, often genetically modified because of the huge cash incentives offered to farmers who grow it. As a result, corn-based ingredients are present in a great majority of processed food products. As a nation, we consume sixty-six pounds per person every year.[21]

Ingredients like maltodextrin, corn starch (usually modified in some way), corn syrup and HFCS can be found in virtually every processed food.[22]

The only way to avoid high fructose corn syrup and other preservatives and chemicals that are toxic to our bodies is to buy unprocessed food. And what is unprocessed food again? Something that's in its *natural* state, and preferable not in a wrapper or a bag: an egg, an apple, a carrot.

Fakers

Fakers are foods that make you think that the food you are eating is something that it's not. They are usually full of synthetic preservatives that make them look pretty and last longer on the shelf. Luncheon meats are a prime example—meats that have had preservatives and food coloring added to them to make them last longer and look more appetizing. Let's take a look at a few more.

BHA/BHT (Butylatedhydroxyanisole)

BHA and BHT are the most common human and pet food preservatives. They are antioxidants that protect fats and oils from becoming rancid and developing an off-flavor. They help food companies fake the quality of the food you are eating by preserving it beyond its natural life. Hmmm … I'm not sure I want my kids eating this either!

Despite the fact that safe alternatives are available, these preservatives are widely used by food manufacturers. Many research studies indicate BHA and BHT are carcinogens, which means they can cause cancer.[23]

BHA and BHT are often found in the following common food items:

- *Potato flakes*

- *Dry breakfast cereals*

- *Enriched rice*

- *Foods containing animal fats and shortening*

- *Chewing gum*

- *Potato chips*

- *Vegetable oils*

A surefire way to keep BHA and BHT out of your kids' diet is to buy nitrate-free (see Nitrates, below) sandwich meats like ham, turkey or bologna and to buy nitrate-free or natural bacon as well. These are readily available at most stores now. Some of my favorites are Applegate Farms and Pederson Farms. They provide wonderful hormone- and nitrate-free pork products, beef, chicken and turkey hot dogs, cheeses and other gourmet sliced meats. Pederson Farms even has Little Smokies for parties, patty breakfast sausages and links as well as bacon, ham, Canadian bacon, turducken, bison and stuffed chickens. If you check your grocery store or ask your butcher, there are also often many local producers that will offer nitrate-free meats.

Nitrates/Nitrites

Nitrites are additives used to give cured meats such as ham, bacon and hot dogs their pink color, to prevent the growth of bacteria that can lead to botulism and other food-borne diseases, to preserve products so they can have a longer shelf-life and give the cured flavor that we have come to expect in certain prepared meats.

Products labeled "uncured" contain nitrites derived from celery powder and sea salt, which is a naturally derived preservative. However, they do not contain *synthetic* sodium nitrite which is much more dangerous for our kids. When the nitrates in the celery powder and sea salt react with lactic acid they are converted into nitrites. Without these natural nitrites uncured pork or beef products would be gray. So you can see the attraction to consumers. Who wants to eat gray meat, especially if they are told that the nitrites are harmless?

Unfortunately, many conventional food companies use *synthetic* sodium nitrite to cure their products. Industrial sodium nitrite is allowed to contain *residual heavy metals, arsenic and lead.*[24] Coincidentally, heavy metal poisoning is thought to be one of the key contributors to the rapid rise in autism.[25] While some may say "nitrites are nitrites," those derived from celery juice and sea salt are clearly different.[26]

The nitrosamines that grow in cured meat from nitrates have been linked to cancer, chromosomal damage, birth defects and pregnancy loss in laboratory animals.[27]

Nitrates/nitrites are commonly found in the following meats, unless you specifically buy nitrate-free:

- *Luncheon meats like bologna or ham*

- *Bacon*

- *Hot dogs*

- *Any dried meats, like the beef jerky you might find in a convenience store*

Sulfites

Sulfites are also food additives that help preserve freshness. Sodium sulfites were commonly added to fresh produce and meats to help retain color until reactions of varying severity began to happen, prompting the FDA to take action. After a lengthy investigation into the possible health risks of sulfites, the FDA restricted their use in 1986, disallowing their use in fresh produce or foods containing vitamin B-1, which is destroyed by sulfites. Producers of foods containing sulfites are, however, required to declare the presence of sulfites in quantities greater than ten parts per million on the label.

Sulfite sensitivities can manifest in symptoms as mild as a headache or as severe as anaphylactic shock, and they can occur within fifteen to thirty minutes after ingestion. Most reactions are mild, resulting in wheezing or respiratory irritation, but severe symptoms can include a narrowing of the airways and difficulty breathing and emergency treatment may be required. Most reactions are of a respiratory nature, but symptoms of nausea, diarrhea and abdominal pain have also been reported.[28]

Sulfites are most commonly found in wine, unless labeled otherwise. The good news is, there are now some great labels like Sterling and Bonterra that offer organic wines at a very reasonable price. Here are some other foods to watch out for that usually contain sulfites:

- *Molasses*

- *Dried Fruit*

- *Pickled onions*

- *Sauerkraut*

- *Grape juice*

- *Shrimp*

- *Muffin mixes*

- *Bottled lemon and lime juice*

- *Grapes*

Artificial Food Coloring
(Blue #1, Blue #2, Yellow #6, Red #2, Red #40 and more!):

For many decades, artificial food coloring has made it possible for big food companies to fake the "natural color" of processed foods. Parents and health experts have been aware of the side effects of artificial colors on children for years, but until recently the US Food and Drug Administration has stayed uninvolved in their use and regulation.

Under pressure from activist groups and concerned parents nationwide, the FDA was recently forced to take a closer look at the harmful effects of artificial coloring and food dye on children's health.

Parents have connected several disturbing childhood behaviors with the ingestion of artificial colors, specifically mood swings, hyperactivity, problems with concentration and the inability to control emotions. These symptoms sound like those closely related to a childhood epidemic that's been on the rise: ADHD. Could there be a connection? According to Dr. Kenneth Bock, in his book, *Healing the New Childhood Epidemics*, there is a connection, not only with food coloring, but also with aspartame and MSG, which, as mentioned earlier in this section, are excitotoxins that over stimulate brain cells and can kill them.

Have you noticed that when you give your kids any liquid medicine when they are sick—unless you buy dye-free—that it has a distinct color? These artificial colors and flavors are added to medicine that we give to kids who are already dealing with a suppressed immune system, which only increases their toxic load. Many of these medicines also have artificial sugars in them so they are "sugar-free" (see Aspartame). Artificial colors and flavors can be challenging to avoid. Even white marshmallows have blue food dye to make them look whiter! So what's the answer? Look for dye-free options when buying medication whenever possible to avoid any potentially harmful reaction.

Food dyes—used in everything from M&Ms to sports drinks to Kraft salad dressings—pose risks of cancer, hyperactivity in children and allergies and should be banned, according to a new report by the Center for Science in the Public Interest. A top government scientist agrees, and says that food dyes present unnecessary risks to the public.

The three most widely used dyes, Red #40, Yellow #5, and Yellow #6, contain carcinogens that pose a risk to children. According to the CSPI, another dye, Red #3, has been acknowledged for years by the Food and Drug Administration to be a carcinogen, yet is still in the food supply and being consumed by many of our kids daily. Red #3 is found in canned cherries, baked goods, dairy products and snack foods. For more information on where specific dyes are found, visit http://www.red40.com/pages/other_dyes.html.

Despite those concerns, "each year manufacturers pour about fifteen million pounds of eight synthetic dyes into our foods. Per capita consumption of dyes has increased five-fold since 1955, thanks in part to the proliferation of brightly colored breakfast cereals, fruit drinks, and candies pitched to children."[29]

For more information on what additives and artificial colors and flavors in junk food can do to your kids, check out *The Southampton Shocker*, a study performed in England that has shown evidence of increased levels of hyperactivity in young children consuming mixtures of some artificial food colors and the preservative sodium benzoate.[30]

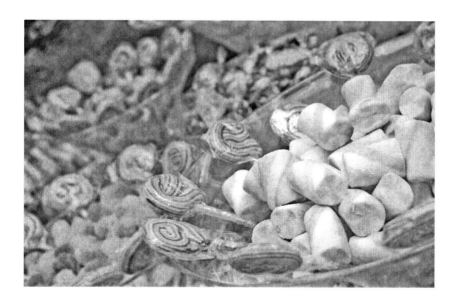

Become Expert Label Decoders

Teaching your children to avoid certain ingredients on nutrition labels can dramatically affect their performance in the classroom, on the sports field and how they behave at home. Following these label-reading guidelines will guide you and your kids to healthy eating habits for life, and you can have fun doing it! My kids enjoy picking up cereal and snack bar boxes at the store to see what the manufacturers are trying to hide with deceptive labeling.

Teach your kids to become expert label decoders too by following these very simple guidelines:

Guideline #1

Avoid products that contain the following:

- *MSG (otherwise known as "Natural Flavors"). You can check the chart for other aliases.*

- *Any artificial food coloring*

- *High fructose corn syrup*

- *Nitrates/nitrites*

- *rBST*

- *Anything that says "partially hydrogenated"*

- *Any artificial sweeteners, like NutraSweet or Equal*

Guideline #2

Avoid food that has more than seven to eight ingredients or contains an ingredient you can't pronounce. These are usually found on the center aisles of the grocery store, where your kids prefer to hang out. Don't get me wrong—this isn't easy! But it will make you stop and think when you see what's going into your kids' food and into their bodies. Once you become aware, you will always be thinking of ways to upgrade.

Example: instead of artificially sweetened, flavored and colored yogurt for breakfast, buy vanilla or plain Greek yogurt and add fresh fruit, nuts and brown sugar or honey!

Guideline #3

Avoid food that's not in its natural state. An egg is an egg is an egg; especially when you make it at home. You can't go wrong with fresh food that hasn't been chemically or physically altered in any way. Remember, stay away from food "substitutes" or fast-food imitations. Example: canned mandarin oranges full of high fructose corn syrup and MSG, versus an *orange*! Which one do you think your child's body prefers?

Guideline #4

Avoid foods that come in fun, highly colored packaging. Remember, what you see is not always what you get. There are very few laws governing what words food manufacturers are allowed to write on boxes and wrappers, so buyer beware. Sugary breakfast cereal boxes that say "Natural" or "Whole Grain" or "16 vitamins and minerals" don't mean much. The 16 vitamins are usually sprayed on, after the cereal has already been totally stripped of all its nutrients. Remember who the target audience is: KIDS! Don't choose a cereal or snack by its cover; read the labels for the truth and explain to your kids *why* you're choosing one over the other. Example: Fruit Loops versus whole grain Cheerios with fresh or frozen berries.

TIP: *Enriched vs. Fortified*

When you read labels for foods such as milk, you will often see the word "enriched." Enriched means that vitamins or minerals have been added to the food. The vitamins and minerals are added to replace the original vitamins and minerals that were lost during the refining process. When a food product, such as cereal, reads "fortified" it means that vitamins or minerals have been added to the food in addition to the levels that were originally found before the food was refined. When foods are fortified, they will have more vitamins and minerals after they are refined than they did before they are refined.

"Fortified" is often misused by companies who produce cereal and fruit drinks. Cereal boxes will often say "fortified with essential vitamins and minerals" but the cereal usually contains high amounts of sugar. (www.mamashealth.com)

Guideline # 5

Avoid genetically modified foods both on the shelves and in the produce section. Remember, non-GMO foods will be organic and have a SKU number that starts with a 9. Non-GMO packaged goods are also easy to spot because your kids can look for the little flower label on front that says non-GMO. There is also a great Non-GMO Shopping Guide app that you can get for your smart phone to help guide you in the store. For more detailed and comprehensive information on GMO's, you can visit www.responsibletechnology.org.

"*If you don't take care of your body, where will you live?*"

—KOBI YAMADA

GMO FOODS TO AVOID
(UNLESS THEY ARE ORGANIC):

- Yellow squash
- Zucchini
- Corn (corn oil as well)
- Canola (canola oil as well)
- Soy (soybean oil, tofu, soy flour, baked goods)
- Cottonseed oil
- Papaya (Hawaiian)
- Rice
- Tomatoes

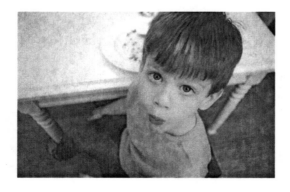

Is your child a green bean or a tater tot?

MAKE A BETTER BAD CHOICE

One summer at camp when my daughter was nine, she was part of a baking exercise in the camp kitchen. The baked good in question was red velvet cake. She told her counselors that cake couldn't be naturally red and when she read the label on the cake box, she confirmed that it did indeed contain red food dye. She chose not to eat the dessert. Does that happen every time? No way. She'll ask for a colored energy drink after a soccer game every chance she gets, so I try to make a better bad choice and buy clear energy drinks for those events. At least they don't contain food dye! The idea is to teach your kids to make a *better* bad choice.

We all know that kids are going to want sweets and other things that aren't the best for their developing brains and bodies. That's a given. The idea is to encourage them to choose something that doesn't fall on the far end of the spectrum! Here are a few examples of better bad choices:

- *Instead of orange flavored soda . . . choose IZZE Sparkling Juice.*

- *Instead of chewy "fruit snacks" . . . choose YummyEarth Organic Gummy Bears.*

- *Instead of cheese puffs . . . choose Pirate's Booty.*

- *Instead of chocolate ice cream . . . choose several squares of dark chocolate.*

- *Instead of store-bought cupcakes with lots of icing . . . bake your own without icing or with homemade icing.*

- *Instead of store-bought cake . . . make an angel food or pound cake with strawberries on the side.*

- *Instead of ordering a popsicle or ice cream at a restaurant . . . order a bowl full of berries with sorbet (or even better, save some money and eat dessert at home).*

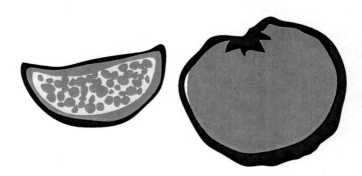

The Kids' Menu Trap

Unfortunately, it's not just food in grocery stores that we have to learn to avoid. Dangerous foods can be found everywhere, including your favorite restaurants. Restaurants are particularly tricky, making it even more challenging for you to present your kids with healthy options.

When dining out with kids, you are often offered a separate "Kids' Menu." This is why most kids grow up believing they are supposed to be eating different foods than adults. They believe that their choices are made up of just a few predictable "kid food" options. This is where the problem starts. Kids are literally being raised to believe that they are *supposed* to eat different food than we are. The brainwashing begins at a very early age.

When was the last time you saw a green veggie offered on a kids' menu? Or whole grain bread? Restaurants know that our kids are used to eating sweet, salty, fatty foods (which make us crave more of them, by the way)—and their kids' menus are designed to cater to this preference. In addition, the portions they are offered are usually way too large!

Let's take a look at a typical kids' menu to get a better idea of what our kids are actually eating:

Pizza

This extremely popular kids' menu option is rarely made with organic or rBST-free cheese, which means our little ones are consuming a load of hormones and antibiotics they don't need. If they choose pepperoni, they're most likely choosing meat that is full of nitrates and/or nitrites, which are seriously harmful preservatives. Unless the tomato sauce is organic or even homemade—which is extremely unlikely—they are eating a vegetable that is at the top of the Dirty Dozen list for pesticide-laden veggies. And the cheese and sauce is likely served on white dough that's been stripped of all its nutrients and probably even had gluten added to it for flavor. Pizza is also one of the hardest things for your body to break down because the combination of dough (gluten) and cheese (casein) wreaks havoc on your child's digestive system and blood sugar. This is even more true if they are diabetic.

BEWARE OF THE REFILL TRAP

In a world of 44-ounce sodas and kids' menus, beware the refill trap in restaurants. It's very easy to lose sight of how many refills you or your child have had of your sugary drink and in no time at all you've consumed your daily recommended amount of calories. If you do decide to treat yourself or your child to a sugary drink, let the waiter know up front that you are not interested in any refills and ask him please to not refill your child's drink as well, unless it's with water. P.S. Water refills don't have *any* calories, so drink up!

Mac n' Cheese

Noodles with cheese sauce is a childhood classic, but it's also one of the worst offenders. Most mac n' cheese is made with artificial food dye in the cheese sauce and highly processed white noodles. The cheese powders used in mac n' cheese usually include dehydrated cheese (pasteurized milk, cheese culture, salt, enzymes), whey, partially hydrogenated soybean oil, whey protein concentrate, lactose, maltodextrin, salt, sodium phosphate, citric acid, lactic acid, yellow #5 and yellow #6—all of the things we are trying to avoid! Luckily, for moms who don't always have time to cook there are many organic versions available now, which at least changes how kids eat at home. Annie's makes a large variety of mac n' cheese options as does Whole Foods 365 brand, and even Kraft has jumped on the bandwagon.

Hamburger

This kids' menu staple is usually made from meat that is not natural or organic (and sometimes barely meat!), which means the meat is full of antibiotics, hormones and pesticides, not to mention red food dye or other sprayed on chemicals to keep it looking "fresh." This "hamburger" is also usually served on a white bun made with high fructose corn syrup and other harmful preservatives. Did I mention the ketchup? Yet another way to add empty calories and toxins to your child's diet. Your best bet is

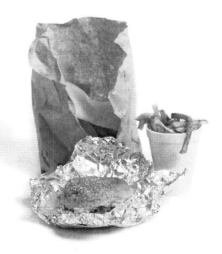

to keep your kids away from red meat when eating out, as commercial meat is one of the worst culprits.

Hot Dog

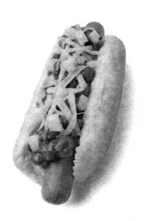

If a kids' menu printed the ingredients of the average hot dog, would you still order it for your child? Here's what you're not seeing: In addition to the pork and beef, hot dogs often contain corn syrup, large amounts of sodium, monosodium glutamate (MSG), sodium diacetate, (for food flavoring and to maintain pH), sodium erythorbate (a food additive), red dye #40, red dye #6 and sodium nitrate. The ketchup that usually accompanies hot dogs is most often made with red food dye and high fructose corn syrup and it's served on a highly processed white bun that turns into glue once it hits your gut. Eating lots of processed meats like hot dogs has been linked to an increased risk of cancer. Part of that risk is probably due to the additives used in the meats, namely sodium nitrite, MSG and red food dyes. How many of you are having an aha moment as you remember your child feeling sick the last time you went to a ball game?

Chicken Nuggets

Some of the more frequently visited fast-food restaurants have over thirty ingredients in their chicken nuggets and tenders. Here are a few of the ingredients you can find: dimethylpolysiloxane, an antifoaming agent made of silicone, also used in Silly Putty and cosmetics; tertiary butylhydroquinone or TBHQ, which is a chemical preservative and a form of butane (lighter fluid). One gram of TBHQ can cause "nausea, vomiting, ringing in the ears, delirium, a sense of suffocation and collapse," according to *A Consumer's Directory of Food Additives*. Five grams of TBHQ can kill you.[31] I don't know about you, but after I read this I decided it wasn't worth it.

Fries

Most French fries are made from genetically modified potatoes. They are often full of salt and deep-fried in hydrogenated oil (think high cholesterol, heart disease, obesity, cancer) and most possibly made from GM soy. And don't forget the ketchup, one more way to add HFCS, sodium, MSG and red food dye to an already killer (literally) meal. Did I mention that they are everywhere?

Shirley Temple, Lemonade, Fruit Punch or a Soft Drink

Drinks designed for kids are usually made with high fructose corn syrup from genetically modified corn, which is grown with massive amounts of pesticides. Drinks that include grenadine and red cherries are loaded with red dye. Some child-themed beverages even contain aspartame. Come on moms, just say "no!" A little lemonade or cranberry juice mixed with club soda is fine for a treat, and served in a cup holds an age appropriate amount for their tiny tummy, like 4-6 ounces.

But giving your six-year-old a 20-ounce cup of soda just doesn't make sense!

This may seem like a lot of information to take in at once—even scary and overwhelming. After I learned all of this, I was afraid to let my kids eat at some of the restaurants we chose. But I learned how to integrate healthy eating into everyday living. What do you do when there are no good choices? Well, you just make a better bad choice: grilled, not fried; fruit, not fries; and wheat not white.

HINTS FOR CHILDREN:

Make an iced tea out of hibiscus flower. (Available in any grocery store.) Mix with lemonade or orange juice in the summer to make it pink. Hibiscus is full of antioxidants and has a cooling effect on the body. Another way to create that pink color that kids love is to add raspberry juice to any fruit drink.

Make smoothies out of organic berries (thin skinned berries are in the list of the dirty dozen so buy organic), fruit juice, banana and yogurt. No sugar is necessary if the juice is naturally sweet. The banana also contributes sweetness and fiber. Add craisins, raspberries and dried currants to muffins.

The "Our Family" Motto

Submitting to the demands of your child may turn him or her into a selfish, entitled adult. But more importantly, allowing your child to make big decisions is dangerous, especially when it comes to food. Kids do not have the knowledge or experience to make healthy choices for themselves. A five-year-old is incapable of making wise nutritional decisions when you are at the food court in the mall, just as she is incapable of understanding why it's more important to be running around outside than playing Wii for four hours straight inside. To quote Dr. Sears, "Kids will choose taste over nutrition, unless they are programmed otherwise."[32] Children are by design impulsive and self-focused. And they are driven by an innate selfishness to get what they want regardless of what the physical consequences may be.

As parents, it's our job to teach our kids the right way to eat. This responsibility doesn't fall to school, government or anyone else. We are the ones who buy the groceries; we also vote with our wallet. We are the ones who they see driving the car into the fast-food drive-thru or maybe they see fast-food wrappers on the floorboard of our car. We are the ones who take them to a restaurant and then cave in to their relentless whining for pizza because we want to avoid a noisy scene. And we are the ones who will be responsible when our child becomes a statistic at eighteen, with Type II diabetes, high cholesterol or insulin dependency. One out of three kids born in the year 2000 will be insulin dependent by adulthood.

As parents, we have an obligation to give our kids the necessary tools to be happy, healthy and successful in life. And this starts with eating habits that foster long-term wellness.

A great way to instill the "Our Family" motto is with food. When kids complain about what's on their plate, my answer is always, "In our family, this is how we eat." (Just make sure you're eating it too, or you will lose all credibility!) Kids look to their parents and to their older siblings to set an example. If you don't practice what you preach with them, you've lost before you even started. This is especially true when it comes to choosing real food over fast food choosing water over soft drinks ("liquid candy"), making home-cooked meals and exercising on a regular basis. We will talk about this more in depth in the next section of the guide.

It's easy to upgrade the quality of your kids' menu without a whole lot of complaining from the peanut gallery, whether you're eating at home or eating out.

Below are some examples of new and improved Our Family Kids' menus.

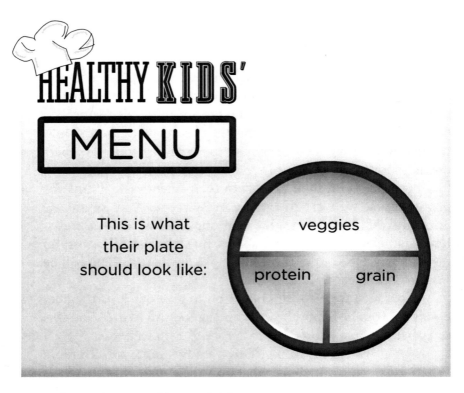

HEALTHY KIDS'

MENU

This is what their plate should look like:

veggies

protein   grain

"Our Family" Pizza

Make a homemade pizza with rBST-free cheese, nitrate-free pep-peroni and organic red sauce. These ingredients are super easy to find at any grocery store. Costco carries both organic pasta and pasta sauce. Serve it with some carrots and fruit or a salad, and presto, you've gone from toxic to terrific! You can even use mini whole wheat tortillas, English muffins or pita bread for personal pizzas and let the kids add veggies like sliced bell peppers, mush-rooms, cauliflower and onions.

For premade healthy pizzas, try Amy's brand (www.amys. com), Annie's, which now has an organic frozen rising crust pep-peroni or spinach and cheese pizza, or Kashi (www.kashi.com). We like to add our own toppings to personalize the experience.

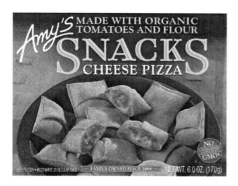
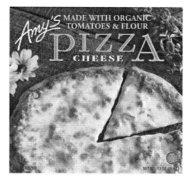

"Our Family" Mac n' Cheese

Homemade or store-bought mac n' cheese is fine from time to time, as long as it is part of a balanced dinner served with steamed asparagus, green beans, broccoli, snow peas or a green leafy salad. Even if you don't use organic cheese, your kids will be getting a much healthier meal with less sodium, no MSG and a large variety of multicolored veggies. Kids also love broccoli, which you can buy in large bags at Costco and melt some cheese on the side for dipping if they like it that way. Try not to pour it on top of the vegetables as you tend to pour a lot more than they would usually eat and it keeps them from really learning to taste and grow accustomed to the food.

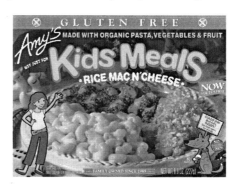

"Our Family" Hamburger

Whenever possible, buy natural, hormone-free hamburger meat and organic ketchup, which doesn't include high fructose corn syrup or red food dye. These are very easy to find now in most grocery and superstores like Sam's Club or Costco. If that's not in your budget, even cooking regular hamburger meat at home is a better choice for your family than getting a fast-food burger full of additives like soy and food coloring. If you do order a hamburger when you eat out, always ask for a whole wheat or whole grain bun—you might be surprised. Or, even better, you can encourage your kids to eat the burger without a bun and add fruit and veggies to the order. Sometimes, at home, I "forget" to buy hamburger or hot dog buns and serve brown rice. Keep in mind that it's important to encourage your kids to try new foods both at home and when you eat out. If we have a week where I know our schedule is going to require us to eat out more than once, I talk with the kids ahead of time and explain that they may choose a hamburger once that week, but not twice. In addition, if they've already had one at school that week, then I ask them to choose something else. I try to limit the red meat intake as much as possible, and at home when we do cook it I love to make "sliders," (mini-burgers), so the amount of meat they are eating is smaller, and then we fill up the plate with other yummy foods.

"Our Family" Hot Dog

Buy organic hot dogs or at least nitrate-free or kosher dogs. There are so many healthy options out there in most grocery stores that I love: chicken dogs, turkey dogs and the regular beef hot dog. There are many to check out, but as I mentioned earlier, two of my favorite brands are Pederson Farms and Applegate Farms. Serve it with a whole-wheat bun, organic ketchup and some homemade coleslaw or diced veggies for a balanced lunch. Another fun variation on this for lunch or even breakfast is to serve kielbasa, bratwurst or another German sausage (which all come in hormone-free versions). They can be served on a whole-wheat bun or with homemade red potato salad (vinegar-based which is healthier) and you can even add sauerkraut or grilled onions. This is another way to add some variety to your child's diet, introducing them to another kind of "hot dog." In fact, many ballparks already offer bratwurst as an option.

"Our Family" Chicken Nuggets

When you order a chicken nugget from a fast-food restaurant, chicken is far from the only thing you get. The average fast-food or restaurant prefrozen nugget contains: *some* white boneless chicken, MSG, salt and many chemical additives and fillers.

Most are then battered and breaded with: bleached wheat flour, a few "spray on" vitamins and more chemicals. They are then fried in vegetable oil: GM canola oil, GM corn oil and hydrogenated soybean oil with TBHQ and citric acid added to preserve freshness. Are you getting the picture? *None* of these provide any of the nutrients our kids' brains and bodies need to grow and perform in school and on the athletic field.

Most nuggets also contain several completely synthetic ingredients, from a refinery or chemical plant. These chemicals are what make modern processed food possible, by keeping the food materials in them from going bad or looking strange after months in the freezer or on the road. The most alarming ingredient in most nuggets is tertiary butylhydroquinone, or TBHQ, an antioxidant derived from petroleum that is either sprayed directly on the nugget or the inside of the box it comes in to "help preserve freshness."[33]

According to *A Consumer's Dictionary of Food Additives*, TBHQ is a form of butane (i.e., lighter fluid) the FDA allows processors to use sparingly in our food. This is definitely a good thing since ingesting a single gram of TBHQ can cause "nausea, vomiting, ringing in the ears, delirium, a sense of suffocation and collapse. Ingesting five grams of TBHQ can kill."[34]

When we do decide to go with a chicken nugget, strip or tender on a night where I am just too tired to really cook, my kids prefer Bell and Evans chicken tenders and strips. They even provide a gluten-free version. Applegate Farms and Coleman Naturals also make a great organic nugget. No TBHQ, genetically modified soy or other undesirable and toxic additives. If you're feeling a bit more energetic, you can easily bake your own made with whole wheat breadcrumbs or panko (Japanese breadcrumbs).

Just as a reference point, here are the ingredients in homemade fried chicken: bone-in chicken pieces, milk, eggs, flour, canola oil, salt and pepper. For a healthier version, cut the canola oil and just bake them!! This is actually an easy dish the kids can help with as well.

"Our Family" Fries

If you can't go without fries, make them at home. Sweet potato fries are a great substitute as long as you don't cover them with chili and cheese! You can buy them precut in the freezer section or make them yourself. You can also make crispy, tasty homemade fries in the oven. Serve them with organic ketchup or a brand that doesn't use high fructose corn syrup or red food dye. Heinz has a great one that they sell at Costco in pairs in bulk sizes; so do Randall's, Wal-Mart, Trader Joe's, Organicville Foods and Whole Foods. Remember: children have to be exposed to a new food ten to fifteen times before their palates can accept it. If your child is accustomed to regular fries and is resistant to switching over, don't give up! We'll talk about that more in the next section and give you the tools you need to make the necessary changes without completely upsetting the balance in your home.

"Our Family" Shirley Temple

If your kids choose a sweet or semisweet drink for dinner, remind them that they are choosing that beverage as their dessert. In my house there is no such thing as a soda or juice for dinner and then a dessert as well. I love to see the girls talk amongst themselves, debating which they'd rather have. Keep in mind that there is no reason to offer a sweet drink or dessert more than once or twice a week. If your kids are anything like mine, I'm sure they're getting more than their fair share of desserts and juice at school and at friends' houses afterwards. They've fallen into the mind-set that they need a dessert every night, or at least they try to convince us that they do.

As we talked about earlier, if your kids do choose juice or soda, make a better bad choice and mix juice with sparkling water to cut the sugar, or go for "spa water" where you add slices of lemon, lime or cucumber to make the water look pretty as well as give it a unique flavor. You can easily do this whether you are at home or in a restaurant.

MAKE A CHOICE: JUICE OR DESSERT

This is a big one in our house. I make it very clear to my kids that juice is a dessert, and that they are going to have to choose one or the other if I decide to allow it that day. If they decided to go for a lemonade or a sports drink at their softball game, remind them that this means no juice or dessert later in the evening, even if you are going out or attending a birthday or special function. This will help them to realize what sugar really is and help them to control their intake on their own. The thought process is simple for them: if I have **this** soda now then I won't be able to have **that** special dessert for grandmother's birthday later. It's very empowering.

THE GLUTEN EXPERIMENT

Some of you may be wondering why I suggest substituting rice or veggies for the hamburger or hot dog bun on occasion. I wanted to explain to my girls what happens in your body when you eat wheat flour (like you find in a hamburger bun), so I decided to do an experiment with them. We poured several cups of flour into a bowl, and then we added a few cups of water. I asked them to then try and stir the mixture. Surprise! It was very hard for them to stir it. The "gluten" in the flour had turned our mixture into a sticky, gluey mess. Gluten, by the way, is simply a protein that is formed when wheat flour is moistened and then mixed or kneaded. This sticky mess also forms in your stomach when you eat products with gluten. The gooey mass then has to pass through your digestive tract. It shows the kids how hard gluten can be on your body and how difficult it is for some to digest. Even worse, when you combine it with cheese like on a pizza, it makes it that much harder to pass through your body. Think about the kids—and there are many—who are eating a fast-food sausage biscuit with cheese for breakfast, a burger for lunch, then pizza for dinner, with no veggies or fruit, which are full of the fiber they need to help push the food through their bodies! I hear more and more about children and adults who are unable to pass food through their digestive systems. Everything gets stuck and they have to literally go to the hospital to have it removed. The Standard American Diet (SAD) consists of a disproportionate amount of processed flour, which can wreak havoc on your system. Is this what you want for your child? Teach them moderation and to choose whole grain products without gluten, like brown rice, whenever they get the chance. Their bodies will thank them.

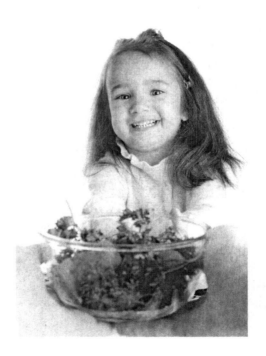

Supplementation

Unless organic, the food that comes out of the ground has been drained of nutrients by herbicides, pesticides and sewage sludge as well as a depleted layer of top soil. We have to find a way to get those nutrients back into our kids. Even though organic fruits and veggies provide 30 percent more nutrients than nonorganic,[35] we can't all afford to buy organic foods, or don't have consistent access to it. Children who eat only the Standard American Diet, are also lacking in nutrients. A diet with minimal fruits and vegetables and lots of highly processed foods can leave kids with a myriad of health issues, like constipation, depression, behavioral issues and lower IQ. This is why supplementation is so important for children today.

By supplementing from a very young age, we can help our kids' bodies stay ahead of the curve. Here is a list of some of the best supplements that you can provide for your child with an explanation of why they help:

Multivitamin

For my young clients, I always recommend a great multivitamin with lots of zinc. Zinc is responsible for sensory development and function, including taste and taste perception. It's also a powerful antioxidant and helps to treat the hyperactive and impulsive aspects of ADHD in children. Zinc aids in regulating brain waves which assist with information processing and helps to lessen distraction, making learning easier. Children who don't eat much and who subsist on the Standard American Diet often become part of a vicious cycle, only eating processed foods, white flour, sweets, breads, pasta, crackers, pretzels, chips, and macaroni and cheese. Sound familiar? These foods are all high glycemic, which means they raise blood glucose, which then quickly increases the demand for insulin production. This increased insulin production depletes their levels of zinc, ultimately resulting in abnormal taste and texture response. If your child's body is low in zinc, many healthy foods like fruits, protein and vegetables can seem repulsive to them, causing them not to want to eat. The smells and textures of foods that might seem typical to us cause an adverse reaction in these children. At the same time, the cravings for unhealthy, processed foods full of MSG and sugar increase. As a result, their health and nutrition level declines rapidly, perpetuating the cycle. By adding in more zinc and slowly introducing new foods one at a time, as well as eliminating highly processed foods, I have found that most children are eventually able to get back on track.

On the flip side, you want to be sure they are not getting too much iron. Iron is important because it carries oxygen to the muscles and organs and increases production of dopamine (dopamine increases alertness and energy). But some popular vitamin brands can be deadly if the dosing is not followed exactly. Look for brands like Nordic Naturals Chewable Berries, Rainbow Light (www.rainbowlight.com) products and Michael's Naturopathic Products for children, preteens and teens. Try to choose multivitamins whose form of iron is carbonyl, a much safer form of iron, rather than ferrous sulfate. Ferrous sulfate has led to deaths from children overdosing. Once again, reading labels is the key to success and good health.

Some vitamins may have ingredients that can cause an allergic reaction in your child.

Make sure to check your children's multivitamin to see if it's free from the following:

- Yeast and wheat gluten
- Soy protein or other derivative
- Milk and/or dairy
- Sodium, starch and corn
- Artificial colors (food dyes), preservatives and artificial flavorings

Remember: you don't want to give your children too much sugar in the form of a multivitamin. Make sure it tastes good enough for them to want to eat it, but it also should contain less than 1 gram of natural sugar per serving.

Essential Fatty Acids

Our bodies don't produce all twenty-five essential fatty acids that they need on their own, so we need to find an alternative source to get the ones they don't make, omega-3s and 6s, into our kids' bodies. They are definitely not getting them from food unless they are big fish eaters, love flaxseed oil, or pumpkin and sunflower seeds, and eat the heck out of walnuts and dark green leafy vegetables. As Americans on the SAD diet, most of us have an unnaturally high consumption of omega-6s in our diet today and need to balance it out through consumption of more omega-3s. Omega-6s are found in many foods that we eat like salad dressings and other oils found in snack bars or oils that we cook with like corn, peanut, poppy seed, safflower, canola, sesame, soy and sunflower oil. The perfect ratio of omega-6:omega-3 is for our brains and bodies to be in balance is 2:1 or 3:1. For most American, it's more like 6:1, which is why we need to add more EFAs to our diet in the form of supplementation. Remember, nutrition plays a unique role in balancing the biochemistry of the body and the brain.

Where Can I find Essential Fatty Acids

- *Fatty/oily fish like sardines and mackerel*

- *Shellfish*

- *Flaxseed (great to sprinkle in waffles or pancakes) or flaxseed oil*

- *Hemp seed or oil*

- *Soy (make sure it's organic or it will be genetically modified!)*

- *Organic canola oil (great for sautéing or stir fry, also needs to be organic or it will most likely be GM)*

- *Pumpkin and sunflower seeds*

- *Walnuts and walnut oil*

- *Wheat germ*

- *Green leafy vegetables*

TIP:

Buying fish can be confusing! There are so many options, so I will give you two tips to remember to simplify things: look for size and the way the fish was raised. The larger the fish, the higher they are on the food chain, which makes them potentially more toxic. So when in doubt, go for the smaller fish. Secondly, always choose wild over farm-raised fish to avoid fish raised on GM corn in crowded, unsanitary conditions.

Omega-3s

There are many health benefits of omega-3 fatty acids. Research shows strong evidence that the omega-3s EPA and DHA can boost heart health and lower triglycerides. And there are studies showing that omega-3 fatty acids may help with other conditions—rheumatoid arthritis, depression and many more. Omega-3s are also thought to play an important role in reducing inflammation throughout the body—in the blood vessels, the joints and elsewhere. Better yet, for kids with ADD and ADHD, omegas calm upset brains and hyperactive inflammatory systems.

There are several types of omega-3 fatty acids. Two crucial ones—EPA and DHA—are primarily found in certain fish. Plants like flax contain ALA, an omega-3 fatty acid that is partially converted into DHA and EPA in the body.[36]

Fish, krill and plant oil supplements are all good sources of omega-3 fatty acids, so you can't go wrong with any of them. They come in capsule form and chewables as well as liquid to accommodate all ages. The best part is, you can throw it into a smoothie for kids and they have no idea it's even there!

Omega-3s:

- Play a key role in infant growth and brain development

- Are essential to the building and structure of cell membranes, brain and retina

- Play an important role in the production of hormones that control reproduction, hunger and response to stress

- Have antiviral benefits

- Help to relieve depression and improve mood

- Help to prevent or manage asthma (I have seen this first hand with my daughter)

- Can rapidly reduce symptoms of ADD, ADHD and bipolar disorder (Dr. John Ratey, *Driven to Distraction*)

- Stimulate the immune system and fight off inflammation, which studies now show is the root cause of most disease

One of my favorite brands of omega-3s is www.nordicnaturals.com.

Another alternative to fish or krill oils, which are not always desirable to children, is a plant-based oil like BodyBio Balance oil (www.bodybio.com), made from organic sunflower and flax oils. It has the perfect 4:1 ratio of omega 6:3 and kids might prefer this as there is no fishy taste since it's plant based.

This may also be a more desirable choice as most fish today are contaminated with mercury and other industrial chemicals that biomagnify—travel up the food chain—and are then eaten by us.

Probiotics

These days, excessive antibiotic and prescription drug use has made probiotics extremely valuable to both children and adults. Probiotics help to balance the billions of good and bad bacteria that live with us constantly in our intestinal tract. This balance of bacteria in our gut is what keeps us healthy, since over 70 percent of our immune system can be found in our gut (which is also now called the "Second Brain.")[37]

Probiotics

- *may prevent problems in the gut, which are linked to brain disorders like depression, which is on the rise among young people;*

- *may help with absorption of nutrients and digestion of food, which can be thrown off by antibiotics, oral steroids and other prescription medication as well as many of the toxic chemicals we eat daily that are added to our processed foods; and*

- *may help prevent allergies.*

WHAT UPSETS THE BALANCE OF GOOD VS. BAD BACTERIA IN OUR GUT?

When the bad bacteria in the gut outnumber the good, it's called **gut dysbiosis**. Much of the food we consume daily, the antibiotics we give our kids every time they get a cold or an ear infection and other things we ingest with our food like pesticides and preservatives upset the healthy balance in our gut, making it hard for our bodies to fight off other things like yeast infections, allergies and other more serious illnesses. For more information on this, check out Beth Lambert's book, **A Compromised Generation** or the website at www. epidemicanswers.org.

Good bacteria is thrown out of balance by the following factors:

- Antibacterial ingredients, like triclosan, found in many hand sanitizers, toothpastes and soaps. Our world is too clean! All of this cleansing is causing an imbalance in our bodies. Stick with regular soap and water, it works just as well. A US FDA advisory committee has found that the household use of antibacterial products provides no benefits over plain soap and water, and the American Medical Association recommends that triclosan not be used in the home, as it may encourage bacterial resistance to antibiotics. Triclosan is linked to liver and inhalation toxicity, and low levels of Triclosan may disrupt thyroid function. (*www.ewg.org*). For healthier alternatives to hand sanitizer, try EO brand sanitizers, Clean Well or just regular soap and water.

- Environmental pollution

- Chlorine in our water that we drink and bathe in every day

- Pesticides, hormones and herbicides in food and prescription drugs

- Prescription and over-the-counter drugs

Since it is impossible for us to avoid these things in our environment all of the time, we need to give our body and gut a boost. A daily probiotic can work wonders, especially if your child is about to take a round of antibiotics, which can kill off the good bacteria as well as the bad. When this happens, it can lead to more illness because the medication kills off all the good bacteria, leaving none left to fight off any invaders—the fancy term for this condition is *immune dysregulation*.

You can get similar benefits from drinking some of the great kefir yogurts available today. They're full of drinkable probiotics. Check out lifeway.net for the different flavors available. Spoonable yogurt is also packed with probiotics. Thick, luscious Greek yogurt is a satisfying snack or dessert. Stoneyfield Farms (Oikos Organic Greek Yogurt), Yakult and Fage make delicious varieties. I also love to use plain Greek yogurt as a sour cream substitute. You can't tell the difference and the health benefits are so much better—plus there's almost no fat!

But it's not enough to rely on food sources for the amount of probiotics our bodies actually need. One of my favorite probiotic supplements is from www.bodybiotics.com and they make small capsules as well as chewables for kids. Nikken.com also has great ones for adults and can be ordered through me at www.welch-wellness.com.

QUALITY COUNTS

It's important to purchase quality probiotics or oils to get the most health benefits. Many supplements and multivitamins that you find on the drugstore or grocery store shelves offer little to no nutritional value and are full of fillers. For guidance on which products are of the highest quality, please visit www.welchwellness.com.

Supplements, however necessary, are not a substitute for the real thing. Don't think that because your children begin taking the supplements I recommend that they are not required to eat any fruits and vegetables.

You can supplement all you want, but it's not an either-or situation. The reality is, the best possible form of vitamins and minerals for your kids is going to come from unprocessed seasonal organic food of the highest quality that was grown locally if possible. When individual vitamins and minerals are separated from the food they are naturally part of, we lose much of the intrinsic benefit we would get from eating the food as nature created it. Every part of the plant works synergistically together to give our bodies the maximum benefit. We can't get that from popping a pill.

Join a co-op, start a mini garden, shop sales and do everything you can to get organic, seasonal fruits and vegetables into your children every single day, several times a day. If you can't afford organic, go with conventional and wash them with veggie spray to get the pesticides off as best you can. Help them to make good choices at school by talking about the menu ahead of time. If there are none, send a lunch with them and start trying to effect change in their school. You will be astounded by how rapidly your child's behavior, health and appearance will begin to change when you clean up what they are putting into their mouths.

> When was the last time you saw a green veggie offered on a kids' menu?

What to Eat

So far we have talked primarily about what not to eat. Now let's take a look at what foods are safe and beneficial to feed our children. We have so many wonderful foods available to us today, each with their own incredible vitamins, minerals and healing qualities. Making sure that our kids are eating fruits and veggies all day long is not optional; the benefits they receive from eating this rainbow of foods will last far into their lifetime.

As long as they are clean, washed, fresh or even frozen, we never have to worry about what negative effects organic fruits and vegetables are going to have on our kids' brains and bodies. There are no fakers, tricksters or swindlers. There are no bad choices—unless of course your child has a food allergy.

Eat the Rainbow (See my "Rainbow Recipe" section for rainbow-inspired recipes.)

Think of what a world without color would be like. No more blue skies or vibrant sunsets to delight and inspire us. We are all touched, inspired and comforted by color. When it comes to food, color inspires our appetite so that our body can receive the nourishment they need. Just as male birds are adorned with bright colors in order to attract their mates, the beautiful colors of our fresh fruits and vegetables are designed to tempt us to eat them. Every fruit and vegetable contains particular nutrients specific to that color that our bodies need to stay healthy and perform at their optimum.

The natural colors of vegetables and fruits are visible signs of the nutrients within them. It then only makes sense that if we eat a variety of colorful foods we will be supplying our bodies with the variety of nutrients required to be healthy and strong.

If you picture a rainbow you will see purple next to red and red next to orange. Just as the colors in the rainbow have similar light spectra to the adjoining color, foods that are purple contain some of the same nutrients as red, the adjoining color. And red foods share some of the same as orange and orange with yellow, yellow with green.

Let's take a closer look at the food rainbow.

Favorite Orange and Yellow Fruits and Vegetables

Orange and yellow fruits and vegetables will help keep your children healthy and out of the doctor's office, saving you both time and money. Who doesn't want that? In addition, many of these are naturally sweet, making them more appealing to children.

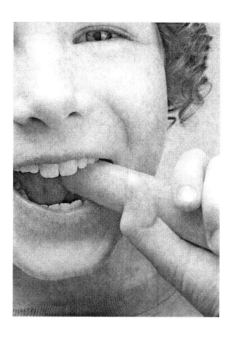

- *Apricots*

- *Bananas*

- *Butternut squash: great for pregnant moms and their babies!*

- *Cantaloupes: strengthen eyes and lungs*

- *Carrots: are sweet with natural sugars that give your kids sustained energy which cookies and candy don't do.*

- *Citrus fruits*

- *Guava: one of the three best fruits and veggies you can eat.*

- *Mangoes*

- *Nectarines*

- *Papayas: are another one of the three best fruits you can eat!*

- *Pears*

- *Peaches*

- *Pineapples*

- *Yams and sweet potatoes: Have a moody teenager due to hormone fluctuation? Or are you hormonal yourself? Try eating yams and sweet potatoes. They are also great for digestive problems in kids.*

- *Yellow apples*

- *Acorn squash*

- *Corn*

- *Yellow tomatoes*

- *Yellow peppers*

- *Yellow squash*

- *Yellow potatoes*

Orange and yellow fruits and vegetables contain the following nutrients:

- **Carotenoids**: *convert to vitamin A, which helps maintain good vision in kids and helps teens fight against acne and eczema.*

- **Bioflavonoids**: *provide calcium and magnesium, which work together to keep kids' bones strong.*

- **Potassium**: *helps children maintain proper fluid levels while participating in sports.*

- **Vitamin C**: *boosts children's immune systems, supports healing and helps the body absorb iron and burn fat. Vitamin C also helps keep children's lungs strong and protects against heart disease.*

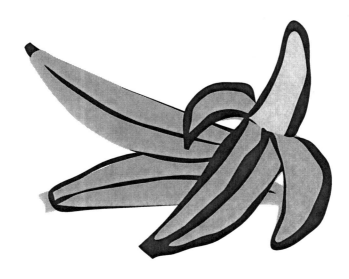

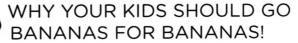

WHY YOUR KIDS SHOULD GO BANANAS FOR BANANAS!

Bananas are

- the most popular fruit in the United States;
- not one of the Dirty Dozen—so they don't need to be organic;
- high in potassium, which prevents cramping during strenuous exercise and strengthens kids bones;
- likely to help your kids relax and sleep more soundly;
- full of serotonin, which keep your kids from being cranky;
- easy to digest—they are an ideal early food for babies;
- a great source of energy—bananas high content of complex carbohydrates supplies energy without crashing later;
- an ideal substitute for sugary snacks— the riper the banana, the sweeter; (Eating a banana can prevent a drop in blood sugar and delay the need for more food.)
- high in vitamin B6, which protect against heart disease and helps to regulate the nervous system; and
- high in fiber and very filling—unlike junk food and sugary snacks—this means your kids won't constantly be saying, "Mom, I'm hungry."

Favorite Red Fruits and Vegetables

Are your kids regular jumping beans when it comes to sitting still and focusing in class? Are you ever stressed out? Vitamin B5, the antistress vitamin will help. It is in red fruits and vegetables and great for helping your kids focus in school and will help all of you deal with stress. Here are some suggestions for red fruits and vegetables to serve to your kids:

- Red apples
- Cherries
- Cranberries (fresh and dried)
- Raspberries
- Pink grapefruit
- Pomegranates
- Red grapes
- Red pears
- Red currants
- Strawberries
- Watermelon
- Beets

- Hibiscus flowers
- Radishes
- Radicchio
- Red-tipped lettuce
- Red bell peppers
- Red chili peppers
- Red potatoes
- Rhubarb
- Red clover
- Red onions
- Tomatoes (actually a fruit)

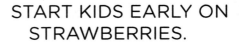

START KIDS EARLY ON STRAWBERRIES.

Strawberries are
- one of the eight best cancer fighting foods;
- sweet tasting and easy to eat;
- appealing to children; and
- easy to eat (try dipping in dark chocolate for special occasions).

Remember: they can cause serious allergic reactions in children, so please don't feed them to your kids before the age of two.

Red Fruits and Vegetables Contain the Following Nutrients:

- **Vitamin B5**: *antistress vitamin, great for helping kids focus in school and supporting every family member through stress.*

- **Anthocyanins**: *powerful antioxidants that help with heart and brain function and fight cancer in the GI tract.*

- **Omega-3 Fatty Acids**: *promote strong HDL cholesterol levels.*

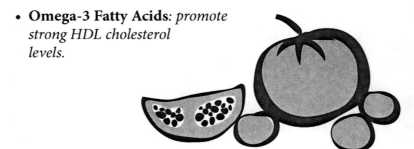

- **Beta carotene**: *converts to vitamin A, which helps maintain good vision and healthy skin.*

- **Vitamin C**: *supports a healthy immune system, aids the body in cellular repair and helps absorb iron.*

- **Vitamin K**: *essential for maintaining healthy bone density and promoting clotting of the blood.*

- **Phytoestrogens**: *help stabilize the menstrual cycle.*

- **Manganese**: *regulates blood sugar and thyroid and aids in calcium absorption, which is essential for building strong bones.*

- **Folic Acid, B6**: *helps alleviate menstrual cycle problems and protects against heart disease and spinal problems with unborn babies.*

- **Antioxidants**: *keep the heart healthy, prevent cellular damage in the body and help soothe inflammation in the body.*

- **B5, Pantothenic acid**: *the antistress vitamin, essential for making hormones, strong red blood cells and antibodies in the body. Most importantly, it detoxifies the body removing harmful pesticides and drugs.*

- **B3, Niacin**: *turns protein, fat and carbohydrate into energy and is beneficial to the heart, skin, lungs, diabetes and arthritis. Note: Because these vitamin Bs are water soluble they are continually flushed out of our bodies in urine. We need to resupply our body daily with these vitamins.*

- **Copper**: *helps build hemoglobin and keeps bones, blood vessels and nerves healthy.*

- **Magnesium**: *builds strong bones by aiding in the absorption of calcium, relaxes the muscles. Excellent for relief of growing pains!*

- **Iodine**: *essential for function of the thyroid glands.*

Favorite Green Fruits and Vegetables

Green vegetables are key to our general health and wellness and are essential for young children as well. Remember Popeye and his cans of spinach? Rich in anitoxidants and high in vitamin C, green veggies like spinach, kale and broccoli pack a mighty health punch. In addition, unlike some other veggies that require at least a little cooking, many of these are great raw or almost raw.

Did you know that one cup of broccoli contains as much vitamin C as one orange? Broccoli also helps restore sun-damaged skin, promotes bone growth and boosts the immune system.

Green lettuces are also important for balancing acid indigestion, preventing constipation and colitis and minimizing gout. In addition, the magnesium found in romaine lettuce helps to revitalize muscular tissue, brain and nerve cells.

So make sure to include at least two or three of these in your child's diet every day, and remember: these are habits you're helping them build for life!

> Eating your fruits and veggies raw is the best way for you and your kids to get the most nutritional bang for your buck! For more information about eating raw or even going fully raw, check out the guru of raw food, Kristina at fullyraw.com

Below are some examples of green foods for your kids to enjoy:

- *Green apple*
- *Green grapes*
- *Honeydew melon*
- *Kiwi*
- *Limes*
- *Pears*
- *Artichoke*
- *Asparagus*
- *Basil*
- *Bok choy*
- *Broccoli*
- *Brussels Sprouts*
- *Cabbage*
- *Celery*
- *Cilantro*
- *Fennel*
- *Green beans*
- *Green bell pepper*
- *Green onions*
- *Kale*
- *Lettuce*
- *Oregano*
- *Parsley*
- *Peas*
- *Seaweed*
- *Spinach*
- *Swiss Chard*
- *Thyme*
- *Watercress*
- *Zucchini*

Green Fruits and Vegetables Contain the Following Nutrients:

- **Chlorophyll**: *Green vegetables get their green color from chlorophyll. Chlorophyll raises the hemoglobin count in our bodies giving us more oxygen, which results in more energy and better circulation. Chlorophyll also helps build iron in the body, raises good cholesterol and lowers bad. It also supports the body's ability to cleanse the liver and colon of heavy metals and toxins, which lowers cancer risks. Chlorophyll also helps remove bad odors from the body and breath.*

- **Carotinoid**: *helps protect the health of the eye (the orange pigment is just hidden by the large amount of chlorophyll).*

- **Manganese**: *regulates blood sugar and thyroid and aids in calcium absorption, which is essential for building strong bones.*

- **Calcium**: *for strong bones.*

- **Folate**: *critical in preventing neural tube disorders.*

- **Vitamin C**: *aids the body in cellular repair and helps absorb iron. C also boosts children's immune systems, supports healing, helps the body absorb iron and burn fat and helps keep children's lungs strong.*

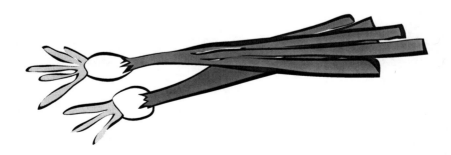

- **Vitamin E:** *is an antioxidant that contains natural tocopherol, which helps support your brain, and cardiovascular and respiratory systems. It also promotes healing.*

- **Iron and copper:** *iron carries oxygen to the muscle and organs and increases production of dopamine. Copper aids in proper growth, strengthening connective tissues, hair, eyes, ageing and energy production.*

- **High in fiber:** *aids in digestion and prevent colon cancer.*

FUN SUMMER SNACK IDEAS FOR KIDS:

Freeze your fruit as a summer treat. A frozen banana, peach, pear or tangerine can be eaten like ice cream. They are rich and creamy making it a healthy delicious dessert. Just pop it in the freezer with the peel on. They are wonderfully refreshing, just like a popsicle without sugar and NO PREPARATION. Add them to smoothies in the blender for icy sweetness. Mango and peach juices are very sweet and less acidic than citrus. Use them also in smoothies and you won't need to add sweetener. When you make fruit salad use fruit juices to keep the fruit from turning brown.

Be sneaky! Look for recipes where you can add bananas, chopped apples, pears, shredded carrots, pureed pumpkin or sweet potatoes to pancakes, muffins and cakes.

Favorite Blue and Purple Fruits and Vegetables (and Black Rice!)

Want your kids to excel in school? Don't forget the blue and purple fruits and vegetables. They protect and support the brain more than any other foods. Here's a list of blue and purple fruits and vegetables that you might enjoy:

- *Blackberries*
- *Black currants*
- *Blueberries*
- *Elderberries*
- *Plums*
- *Purple figs*
- *Purple grapes (and raisins)*
- *Purple cabbage*
- *Eggplant*
- *Purple potatoes*
- *Purple peppers*
- *Black rice*
- *Purple corn*
- *Chokeberries*
- *Black raspberries*

Blue and Purple Fruits and Vegetables Contain the Following Properties:

- *Antioxidants A, E and C, which boost the immune system.*
- *Anthocyanins found in purple corn and chokeberries have been shown to stop cancer cell growth altogether.*

- *Properties that help reduce risk of obesity, reduce belly fat and lower cholesterol.*

- *Blueberries protect and support the brain more than any other fruit. Get out that blender and start making smoothies!*

- *Blueberries help maintain blood sugar and prevent urinary tract infections.*

- *Amazing anti-aging properties.*

- *Anti-inflammatory properties which help fight arthritis.*

- *Brain chemicals that help with prevention of memory loss.*

- *Properties that decrease heart disease by lowering LDL cholesterol.*

- *Improves vision.*

- *Purple fruits and vegetables are important for bone development in children because they improve the body's ability to absorb calcium. They also support their digestive tract.*

- *Lowers risk of cancer in the digestive tract by fighting free radicals.*

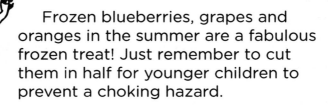

Frozen blueberries, grapes and oranges in the summer are a fabulous frozen treat! Just remember to cut them in half for younger children to prevent a choking hazard.

HELPFUL HEALTH TIP:

Remember to always use veggie wash before eating fruits and vegetables, even if you are buying organic. This will help eliminate toxins on the outer skins of your fruits and vegetables.

IF IT'S WHITE, IT ISN'T RIGHT

We live in a world where the favorite and most common food color for both kids and adults is white: French fries, chicken tenders, hamburger and hot dog buns, donuts, pancakes, pasta, rice, milk . . . you see where this is going. These foods may be tasty, but white is the absence of color, which also means it's the absence of the vital nutrients our bodies need not only to survive, but also to thrive and be healthy.

When White Is Right

White isn't always wrong. White fruits and vegetables have the following beneficial effects:

- *Lower LDL cholesterol*

- *Boost the immune system with strong antiviral and antibacterial properties*

- *Balance hormones*

- *Help reduce risk of colon, breast and prostate cancers*

Favorite White Foods

- *Cauliflower*
- *Onions*
- *Potatoes*
- *Garlic*
- *Oatmeal*
- *Grains*

A woman approached me recently after one of my lectures and told me she was very concerned about her son, who had not grown in a few years and was literally below the growth curve the last time they had been to the doctor's office. The doctor told her not to worry about it, that you couldn't make kids eat.

When she told me what he was eating, there was no surprise: buttered noodles and white bread products. That's it.

As a result of eating a SAD diet consisting only of white food and nothing else, his body was literally so starved of nutrients it could not grow at a time where he should have been growing several inches a year! This should show you the direct correlation between what we put into our kids' mouths (or what they aren't putting in) and their health. What's going to happen to this little boy long term if his parents don't adopt the "Our Family" Motto and empower their child and save his life?

The Benefits of Breakfast

Breakfast is hands down the most important meal of the day for both kids and adults. Not only do children who skip breakfast tend to be overweight, but children who miss breakfast don't perform as well in school, and are not as able to control emotions and behavior due to unsteady blood sugar. Children need a breakfast of complex carbohydrates, like whole grain toast or steel cut oatmeal with nuts and fruit. Make sure to include a protein like a cheese stick, Greek yogurt or a scrambled egg to complement your child's carbohydrate of choice. Top it off with a bowl of fruit (not fruit juice!) and your child's brain and body will be ready to face the day. Even better, when you give them the right serving of complex carbohydrates and healthy protein, their blood sugar will hold steady until lunch time, keeping them from binging on unhealthy carbs, like bread sticks, white bread or crackers in the cafeteria.

Sugary cereals with high fructose corn syrup and food coloring are your enemy. Look for nutritious cereals by examining their labels. Ideally, the cereal will have at least three grams of fiber per serving, three grams of protein per serving and fewer than six grams of sugar. Stay away from fast-food breakfasts like donuts, kolaches or sausage biscuits: they are loaded with saturated fat, gluten, nitrates, sodium and everything else you want to avoid putting into your kids' bodies. Remember: junk food changes their brain and ability to learn.

Finally, don't forget that you can also sneak in veggies like mixed colored bell peppers in the morning as well by adding them to scrambled eggs or an omelette. Being from Texas, I love to add fresh salsa to my eggs. You could even add some avocado or homemade guacamole; avocado is a healthy fat and great for your kids. Give your kids the breakfast they need every day and watch them succeed: they will have more energy, more brain power and feel great.

Eat Whole Foods

Did you know that eating unprocessed, organic food can actually make you skinny? Studies show that the less processed food you eat, the healthier and smaller you are.[38] When you eat processed food with ingredients that are unrecognizable to your body, it holds on to them because it doesn't know what else to do with them! This especially goes for artificial sugars like NutraSweet and Splenda that try to trick your body by making it think it's getting something sweet.

When you open a protein bar or drink a diet soft drink or anything else in lieu of a true meal, are you really eating food the way it was intended to be eaten? Don't we want our kids eating food that's grown out of the ground, without pesticides, hormones and sewage sludge? Ideally, shouldn't the food going into our kids' bodies have the least amount of processing and preservatives possible? Don't we want their food to nourish every intricate part of every intricate system of their precious bodies?

As Michael Pollan says, convenience has turned our food into "edible food-like substances."[39] Combined with all of the environmental toxins we are now exposed to on a daily basis in the air and in our own homes, how much more of this toxic load can our developing kids' bodies take?

You can give your kids real food, food not in a bag or wrapper. Make a decision for your family and stick with it. Be strong! Our modern world has made it pretty easy to take food with us in chilled coolers or soft bags if we need to, so no excuses!

Go Organic

There are many reasons today to buy organic food: depleted nutrient levels in our rapidly vanishing topsoil from rampant herbicide and pesticide use and sewage sludge used to "fertilize plants" just to name a few.[40] However, some foods are not necessarily any safer if you buy them organic, so why spend the extra money? Foods that have thicker, less porous outer skins, like an orange or a pineapple don't have to be organic. But remember, nonorganic foods are more nutrient deficient, so it's critical to supplement your child's diet if they're consuming nonorganic foods and don't eat fruits and veggies with every meal (iceberg lettuce does not count). Later in this chapter I will give you a guide to the Dirty Dozen—which foods are critical to buy organic and which ones are not so critical. This will save you money at the grocery store and also help you to eat seasonally and give your body the nutrients it needs to stay healthy throughout the year.

There has been a lot of buzz over the past several years about eating organic, local and natural foods. There is definitely a lot of information out there, and as moms, sometimes it's hard to sift through it all.

Top Six Foods for Families to Buy Organic

If there are only a few things you can afford to buy organic, make it these six:

- **Milk** *(and other dairy products)—Consider the amount of milk your child consumes from the moment the pediatrician gives you the thumbs-up. You must go organic if you choose to stick with cow's milk to avoid all of the hormones and antibiotics fed to regular cows—not to mention the udder pus from the infections (gross!) which occur from overmilking. Studies show direct links between rBST—the hormones fed to cows to make them produce more milk—and human disease. Personally, I would recommend (organic) rice milk or hemp milk since even organic milk can cause excess mucous production and allergies, eczema, recurrent ear infections and asthma in children. This will also help limit unwanted antibiotic exposure. Considering the US-raised animals we eat* *consumed over twenty-nine million pounds of antibiotics last year according to the FDA, we need to take whatever steps we can to avoid any more unnecessary exposure![41]*

- **Coffee & Tea**—*Our favorite morning beverages are riddled with pesticides and should always be bought organic and filtered through a non-bleached filter. Most of the white ones have been bleached with chlorine. You can find these at Costco, Sam's Club and many other discount shopping clubs.*

- **Apples & Apple Juice**—*Apple juice may be the staple of American children, but apples are one of the Dirty Dozen. Always buy organic apples, applesauce and apple juice for your kids and yourself, if possible, to eliminate taking in the unnecessary pesticides and herbicides sprayed on nonorganic apples, not to mention the sewage sludge in which they have been grown.*

- **Potatoes**—*A double whammy! Most potatoes in the United States are genetically modified (GM) unless they are organic, and are loaded with pesticides. Keep in mind that right now in the United States the law does not require for foods to be labeled as genetically modified, so many of the most popular American foods are genetically modified, thanks to farm subsidies.*

- **Tomatoes**—*With such thin skins, tomatoes are also highly susceptible to herbicides and pesticide, so ketchup should be organic at home, as should pasta sauce and hot sauce if you are making it from scratch. You won't believe the difference in taste either; the organic ones taste fabulous! Branch out and try some organic grape tomatoes as a snack for your kids and introduce them to the yellow ones as well.*

- **Peanut butter**—*Peanuts are heavy with pesticides. Go for the organic peanut butter or another type of butter like cashew butter. There any many brands to choose from now that are easy to find, have less sugar, fewer chemicals and still taste great.*

The Dirty Dozen

Many of us cannot afford to buy everything organic. It would bankrupt most of us. The good news is, you don't have to! However, I do think it's very important to vote with your wallet, and I'd much rather pay for healthy food for my family than doctor visits and prescription medication. The best thing to do is to try to go organic when it's most important, which would be when shopping for foods on the Dirty Dozen list. The Environmental Working Group states that consumers can reduce their pesticide exposure by 80 percent by avoiding the most contaminated fruits and vegetables. Those numbers are nothing to be sneezed at.

The good news: here's a list to help you out. EWG has an iphone app for it now and you can also print it out in a wallet size from www.ewg.org.

"There is really no such thing as junk food— there is just food, and then there is junk."

—DR. MARK HYMAN, MD

EWG's Shopper's Guide to Pesticides in Produce

The Dirty Dozen: The **12 Most Contaminated Fruits and Vegetables.** (Thirty to fifty different pesticides can be found on these items.)

- *Peaches*
- *Pears*
- *Nectarines*
- *Apples*
- *Sweet bell peppers*
- *Celery*
- *Berries*
- *Cherries*
- *Tomatoes*
- *Grapes*
- *Spinach and other greens*
- *Lettuce*
- *Potatoes*
- *Herbs*

Safe to Purchase Conventionally Grown (the least contaminated fruits and vegetables)

- Onions
- Avocado
- Pineapples
- Mangoes
- Citrus
- Asparagus
- Sweet peas
- Kiwi
- Bananas
- Cabbage
- Broccoli

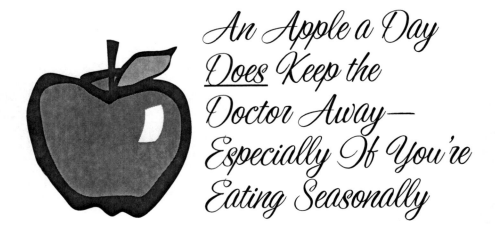

An Apple a Day Does Keep the Doctor Away—Especially If You're Eating Seasonally

What does it mean to eat seasonally? Eating seasonally means that you as a parent are *mostly* buying and consuming the foods that grow naturally in that season. This can be challenging with children who are picky eaters and only like one or two types of fruits or veggies, so it's important to give them a variety from the beginning, as soon as you get the go-ahead from the pediatrician. In a moment, to make your job easier, I will give you a list, naming which fruits and veggies are best for which season. With the advent of modern technology and global agricultural transportation making most fruits and vegetables available year-round, it can be confusing knowing what to buy and when.

In our society today, in a world of on-the-go eating and the fast-food drive-thru, we find ourselves moving further and further away from eating seasonally. Think about it: do you see fast-food restaurants adjusting their menus to serve local and seasonal fruits and veggies? Of course not! So when we eat fast food, we are putting the same foods into our bodies year round, ignoring the changing needs of our bodies with the seasons.

"Having the choice to not eat seasonally has only become an option in the past hundred years or so with all of the conveniences of our modern world. Most people are not even aware that there is a synchronicity between the plants that grow out of the ground and the animals that eat them—including us. The human body has to adapt in a variety of ways to the challenges presented by each season." [42]

So what's the true benefit to eating seasonally? Is there *really* a difference?

HERE'S A SECRET: I learned that the foods from a particular season *can* help the body meet those health challenges associated with that season.

When we get away from eating foods that are most beneficial for a certain season, our bodies can and will fight back. For example, would it make sense to you in the summer when it's warm to eat cooling foods like yogurt and watermelon, or heavy and spicy foods like red meat and salsa?

For example, what are the fruits in season during the winter and cold-and-flu season? Grapefruits and oranges! This is no accident. These foods high in vitamin C are what our kids' bodies need to fight off the numerous germs and viruses surrounding them during this season.

If you are interested in learning more about eating seasonally and the amazing science of Ayurveda, please visit www.joyfulbelly.com or www.banyanbotanicals.com which can help you determine what foods are best for YOU personally in each season.

Now, here is a cheat sheet for the top foods to eat during each season that will help your body combat the weather and specific health issues associated with each season. These foods will also help your body transition into the next season.

Winter

For most of us, winter is the coldest, driest time of the year. This also tends to be the cold and flu season. Since the weather is so dry, our bodies tend to produce more mucous to keep our membranes and tissues from drying out. We don't exercise as much, but our bodies need heavier foods to keep us warm and grounded until we transition in spring. During this time, our bodies need starchy carbs, fats and heavier proteins like you see listed here. Stews, soups, brown rice and meats are ideal for the winter months and kids tend to love them! They are also easy to make as all you need to do is throw several ingredients into a crockpot or slow cooker on your way to work and the meal is ready when you return.

- Chestnuts
- Grapefruit
- Kale
- Leeks
- Lemons
- Cranberries
- Cherries
- Oranges/tangerines
- Radicchio
- Radishes
- Rutabaga
- Turnip
- Potatoes
- Cheese
- Cinnamon
- Garlic
- Cayenne pepper

Spring

In transitioning from winter to spring, your body needs help drying out. The mucous and potential extra fat left over from the winter months are now no longer needed. Now is the time to eat more drying, bitter and astringent foods to help your body transition easily. These foods are lighter and more nutrient dense. Spring is also a time where most of us are able to begin exercising out of doors again, which is key to the drying out process and losing the extra weight your body needed to stay warm in winter. Spring is a time for detox, eating lighter meals and jump-starting your metabolism with the foods here. And don't forget to drink lots of water to flush your system!

- **Asparagus**
- **Avocados**
- **Beans**
- **Carrots**
- **Cherries**
- **Chicory**
- **Chives**
- **Collards and other cooked greens**
- **Fish**
- **Mangoes**
- **New potatoes**
- **Peas**
- **Salads**
- **Seeds**
- **Strawberries**
- **Spring lettuces**
- **Sprouts of all kinds**
- **Snow peas**
- **Watercress**
- **White meat, like pork and chicken**

Summer

For most of us, summer is the hottest season of the year. This is the time where we want to stay away from heavy food and drinks that can slow us down. Hopefully, if our bodies are in tune and not stuck in the rut of the SAD diet, we will naturally crave cold and soothing foods. This is the time of year to eat more raw foods and focus primarily on fruits, veggies and salads like the ones here. You might even notice a reduction in appetite in both you and your kids, which is normal.

- **Bell peppers**
- **Blackberries**
- **Blueberries**
- **Raspberries**
- **Broccoli**
- **Cucumbers**
- **Eggplant**
- **Green beans**
- **Melons**
- **Mint**
- **Okra**
- **Peaches**
- **Pineapples**
- **Plums**
- **Summer squash**
- **Tomatoes**
- **Watermelon**
- **Zucchini**

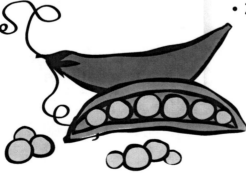

Fall

Fall is a transitional time and can vary dramatically depending on where you live. Here in Texas, we don't really have a fall. It's extremely hot, sometimes even through the month of October. However, there *are* foods that grow specifically to meet the needs of those who live in climates that begin to cool off in September, like the ones listed here. Once again, these foods suit our bodies' needs for the season.

- **Winter squash**
- **Apples**
- **Beets**
- **Brussels sprouts**
- **Cranberries**
- **Figs**
- **Grapes**
- **Mushrooms**
- **Pears**
- **Pomegranates**
- **Pumpkin**
- **Quince**
- **Sweet potatoes**
- **Swiss chard**

(Adapted from *Simple Food for Busy Families* and *Integrative Nutrition*)[43]

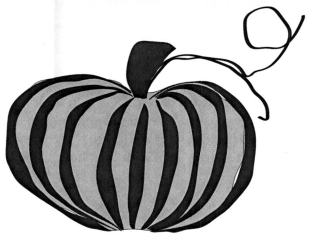

We live on a planet that was designed to give us everything our body needs to be healthy. A hundred years ago, things were simple: people grew and ate what was in season and their bodies responded accordingly. They gathered berries, hunted and fished the animals that were available to them, took them home and ate them. There were no packaged or processed foods. There was also no childhood obesity, heart disease or high cholesterol. There were no food additives or tricky labels to confuse parents and kids.

We now live on a planet where we have access to any fruit or vegetable we could possibly desire any day of the year and thousands of processed foods to choose from. We have deceptive labeling practices and toxic ingredients added to our foods to make them look and taste better as well as last longer on the shelf. This is not nature's design for our bodies. Our bodies were also not designed to withstand GM food, pesticides, herbicides and the thousands of other chemicals that are now part of our food supply.

As a result, we are now a nation with rampant illness on the rise. We need to educate ourselves and our children about the food we eat, teach them what to look for and what to avoid on labels, and teach them what simple supplements to take to strengthen their immune systems. We need to know what's in season and what's important to buy organic so we know what our bodies need; it will also save us money when we are shopping.

We need to teach our kids that when it comes to food, less is more! The fewer ingredients the better, the less packaging the better; the smaller portions the better; the fewer miles the food has traveled to get to you, the better; the less chemicals used, the better.

Once you take these basic steps to understand what to buy to stay healthy, your whole life will change. And so will your child's.

Let's move on and learn how.

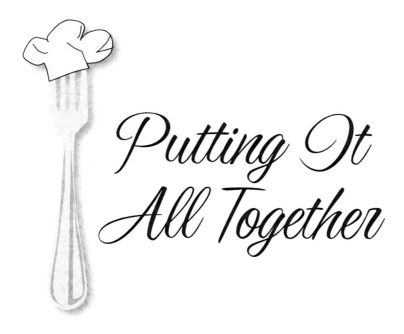

Putting It All Together

By this point in the guide, some of you might feel like it's too late, that you've already damaged your kids. You may feel that there's too much information, and that it's even too hard to turn your family around. You may wonder if it's even worth trying. Well, I'm here to tell you that it's never too late. And it's not too hard. All you have to do is start now. Gradually make changes in the way you and your kids eat at home and on the go and slowly but surely you will educate your children and take back your families' health. You have the power to make these changes. You buy the food, you cook the food, you pay the bill when you go out to eat or cruise through a drive-thru (you need to stop that, by the way!). As parents, it's our job to influence the way our kids eat—no one else's, not the school, not the government or the grandparents. We have an obligation to our kids to give them the tools they need to be happy, healthy and successful in life. To do so we need to integrate simple, effective behavior modification techniques into our kids' everyday lives.

My journey as a mom and health advocate began eleven years ago, the day my first daughter was born. It has been an incredible journey for me, sometimes scary and overwhelming, but also wonderful and rewarding. By seeking better choices for my children, I became more accountable for my family's health and more determined to share what I had learned with other moms.

I have three young girls, ages seven, ten and eleven and have worked with them, from the time they began eating, to consistently expose them to new "real" foods—i.e., foods not found in a wrapper or bag. I tried to resist the media push from commercials and worked to stay strong when my girls begged me to buy "Fun" food while at the grocery store—which most of you know can feel like an impossible accomplishment in the moment. "Fun" food is usually processed and full of food coloring and additives. Think "fruit snacks" or fruit juices that contain no fruit or any other redeeming ingredient. I really love to cook, so when we started having kids I thought, "This will be fun. I get to cook what I love every night for my family and we can all have a tasty and healthy dinner together and everyone will be happy!" Right? Wrong!

Well, I'm sure many of you moms and dads out there got a big kick out of this one. Boy was I crazy! I had no idea what I was in for with three kids under the age of five. I thought that I was doing the best I could to create a happy and peaceful environment, but I

"This is your world... shape it or someone else will."

—GARY LEW

found mealtimes becoming more and more stressful as each year went by with each consecutive child. Though it was challenging, I quickly learned how to parent healthy kids by mastering a good handful of behavior modification techniques, specifically how to manage their *persistance* and *resistance*. This allowed me to keep the peace in our home and my sanity.

When it came to food, there was a battle of the wills in my house every night, starting around 5 p.m. Each child was a different age, with a different palette, and wanted something different to eat at a different time—and was very unhappy if she didn't get it! So, I had to stop and ask myself, "How did this happen? Where did my fun family dinner go?" This was definitely *not* the family life or mealtime experience that I had in mind when we started having kids.

I had lost control of my kids' behavior and their eating habits. Continuing in this way would mean to leave my kids constantly misbehaving, whining and negotiating—leaving me short-tempered, angry, and frustrated. Eventually, we all end up snapping, followed by feelings of guilt. I just didn't want that for me or for my kids every night. I really had to look at what happens when our kids hold the power. I realized that as parents, we become *disempowered* when our kids have control. I knew I had to reclaim control. At first, I didn't think it could happen, or that I could do it or that we could change. As a family we had become so set in our ways and it just seemed like too much work to undo our habits.

There was a part of me that believed it would be easier to stay the same. But, the truth is, it's easier when your kids aren't craving junk food and when they're requesting "real" food instead. Once their diet is clean and they are no longer addicted to sugary snacks and processed foods, they are better focused, better able to listen at home and school, and are able to do what you tell them—and it doesn't have to be hard. But the longer you wait, the more challenging it becomes to change. What I figured out is that short-term pain equals long-term gain. We are going to talk about the resistance and challenges you are bound to face or are already facing with your kids—how they will wear you down and what to do about it.

When I started making these simple changes, within several weeks, I noticed my family and I were both calmer around dinnertime and my kids were more open to trying new foods and less resistant when something green was put on their plate. Now, it is my goal to help you connect the dots and show you exactly how you can do this too, no matter how difficult it may seem at first.

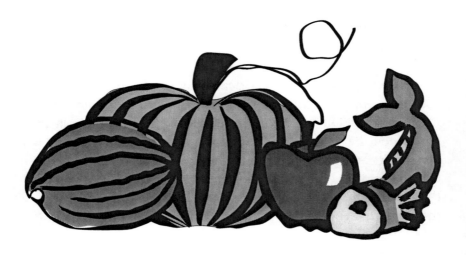

The Top Three Challenges to Getting Your Kids to Eat Right—And Their Solutions

As parents, there are many challenges we face these days when it comes to feeding our kids. After talking to *many* moms, I have narrowed it down to the top three.

CHALLENGE 1:
My Kids Won't Eat Anything Green—or Anything Even Resembling a Vegetable (Well, Maybe a Carrot)

This is the biggest complaint from almost all of my clients, friends and family. Many moms have asked me, "Why did my child eat green veggies when he was a baby and now he won't touch them with a ten-foot pole?" Today, many kids see something green on their plate and they literally run in the other direction, start crying or pitch a fit. I've discovered there are a variety of reasons that children resist green vegetables: texture, flavor or just sheer obstinacy (usually it's the latter because they know they can wear us down). Green veggies cooked the right way can also be difficult to chew at an early age when teeth are still coming in, and even the smallest of kids don't like overcooked food. When you overcook greens or any other vegetable, you also reduce their nutrient density and the health benefits you receive. At any age, we are naturally drawn to crunchiness, so use that to your advantage to serve as many raw veggies as you can!

But the main reason I see children resisting green veggies in my work is that their parents are not serving them consistently from a very early age. Most parents resort to easy finger foods for kids when they advance from baby foods to regular food; think fries and fish sticks.

This goes for eating out as well. Once again, the kids' menu does not offer green veggies, so parents go for what's easy: white, fried, finger foods. This leads to less and less exposure to green vegetables and vegetables in general until you reach a point where the child is now addicted to what he has been given: crackers, puffs, goldfish, fries, white pasta and other food that's easy to serve or carry in a diaper bag.

Usually when their kids are around age four to five, parents start to realize what has happened and panic.

Solution

The solution to breaking the anti-veggie pattern is consistency. You must continue to expose them to green vegetables, and all the others, even after your child is off jarred or homemade baby food and transitioning into whole foods. By serving something green two to three times a day, this becomes your child's "normal" and their palate will grow to accept and love a variety of choices.

Yes, I know it's easier to give them veggies when they are pre-prepared in baby food jars or squeezable bags. I get it. It can also be easy to take steamed, pureed or raw veggies with you once they transition to solid foods. It takes five minutes to steam broccoli or green beans, so let them steam while you are putting together the diaper bag.

Give your kids options by rotating through many kinds of green vegetables: asparagus, sweet peas, snap peas, spinach and

Swiss chard. Try cooking them a variety of ways and try serving them raw. There is no wrong way for your child to eat veggies and some may have a preference due to texture or flavor, raw in a salad or braised and warm. By design, most green vegetables have an astringent or bitter taste, like Brussels sprouts, kale, spinach or bok choy, although some are naturally sweet as well, like green peas. Even though most kids prefer romaine or iceberg lettuce when first testing salads, bitter greens are critical in that they support the liver and help to cleanse our blood and also support the gallbladder. They are also among the most nutrient dense foods available and support the immune system, circulation and can even help clear lung congestion. They should be part of lunch and dinner, every day, for both our children and us.

I prefer to serve the more bitter tasting, cancer-fighting greens like kale, collard or mustard greens and Swiss chard to kids in salads and sauces. When you mix them in with other lettuces like spring mix or romaine, they don't taste as bitter. Another way to serve them and hide the stronger taste is in pasta sauce, either homemade or store bought. The tomato cuts the bitterness and you can mix the sauce with ground turkey, pork or beef. Serve it over pasta or in a meatloaf and the kids will never know the greens are in there.

Remember, you have to expose your child to a particular food fourteen to fifteen times before their palate accepts it. By being consistent, and insisting on the same exposure when you eat out—even if it means bringing the food yourself—you are setting your child up for a lifetime of good habits and good health.

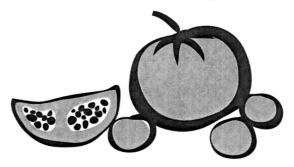

TIP:

Many times, young children will love a certain food and eat it continually, like snap peas and then all of a sudden decide they don't like it anymore. This is normal! Just keep rotating through a variety different veggies even if they appear to have lost interest. Eventually, they will come back to it.

CHALLENGE 2:
It's Easier to Give Them Junk Food Than Real Food Because It's Everywhere

Junk food—food that's not "real" food or "grow" food—is everywhere. It's in our kids' schools, at concession stands at sports games, vending machines, movie theaters, convenience stores, the mall, restaurants and even the fellowship hall at church. It's everywhere your kids are, but you can beat the temptation if you offer healthy food to your children on a regular basis. If you offer junk food to your children, they will eat junk food. Period.

I've had parents and lunchroom and food service workers say to me, "The children should be able to make healthy choices on their own." Come on. What kindergartener or first grade child is going to choose an apple or ham and cheese on whole grain bread over a PB&J on white bread—which is the same as candy, by the way! Or water over chocolate milk? Remember, kids will choose taste over nutrition. Addicts are not in control of their own choices and neither are kids who are addicted to sugary snacks and fast food.

Solution

You can break the junk food addiction cycle simply by saying "no." You have to stop the current cycle you are in and make a decision to change your family's habits once and for all. People want a quick fix and easy answer. Well here it is: just say "no." As I write this book, we are in the throes of softball season for two of my girls. We live at the field. Every week as I watch kids and parents march back and forth to the concession stand, or hear the girls screaming from the dugout for their moms to bring them a blue sports drink, my heart sinks further and further, and I find myself thinking, "Is this the new normal?" (In defense of the concession stand, they do offer one or two healthy food choices like hummus and pretzel sticks and bottled water. However, I have never *once* seen a child walking by with that healthy choice.)

Did you know that the most recent stats show that children who play organized sports are *heavier* than those who don't? [1]

It doesn't take an expert to figure out why, at least from where I sit every week. Are candy, junk food, soft drinks and energy drinks the "New Normal"? Are you willing to accept that? Across all socioeconomic groups, recent statistics show one in seven American kids are obese.[2] When did parents give up and stop telling their kids "NO"? It's a slippery slope with kids: you give an inch, they take a mile, and habits are easily formed before you realize what's happened. Sure, it's hard to say "no" to your kids when they whine, complaining that "everyone else has a sno-cone." So what? Refuse to be the "New Normal." Stand up for your children and their health and teach them while you have the chance. I'm not saying the occasional ICEE or sno-cone is going to kill them—if you do give in, clear flavors are a better choice than red or blue—but let's face it, it's not just occasional any more, it's the new normal. Make a choice to break the cycle. Don't be normal.

Once you have the resolve to say "no," then you can begin to break unhealthy existing habits and establish new, healthier patterns in your family. Have a plan for each location before you go. Think through what challenges you might face before you get there. What snack is your child going to ask for at baseball practice? How will she be tempted at the movies? What will you say when your kids try to eat three cupcakes at a birthday party?

Be prepared. Once you develop a plan of attack and start implementing it, you won't feel as intimidated to say "no."

TIP:

Want to keep down calories as well as cost at the theater? Eat before going to the movies— or at least skip the butter on the popcorn. The same strategy goes for birthday parties: fill 'em up on the good stuff ahead of time and they won't want as much junk at the event. And when buying treats, ask for a smaller size. Believe me, your kids will notice. My kids used to ask me why I order a junior cup when we go out for frozen yogurt. My answer: "Because that's all my body needs." Over time, they started to order in the same way because they realized my body is much larger than theirs, so if I only need a junior size, then why would they need anything larger?

CHALLENGE 3:
Organic Food and Sometimes Even Fruits and Veggies Are Outside of Our Family's Grocery Budget

Many families feel that they can't justify the cost of fruits and veggies to feed their kids, and that it's less expensive and more convenient to drive through and pick up a fast-food meal for lunch or dinner, or even both.

We live in a time where everyone has to be budget-minded and watch their spending. But this shortsighted approach to feeding your kids is going to end up costing both your family and our country more in the long run.

If you look at the price of fast food and what you're actually getting nutritionally—which is almost nothing—for what you're spending, and think about what you're going to have to pay in medical bills down the road, skimping on "real" food is not a good deal! Personally, I would rather spend my money on good food for my kids than on doctor visits and prescriptions or over the counter medications.

Solution

According to the National Institute of Health, we have spent around $113.9 billion due to obesity and overweight related diseases.[3]

Eric Schlosser, author of *Fast Food Nation*, says annual health care costs in the United States stemming from obesity approaches $240 billion.

The good news is, we can turn this around. How, you ask? By making better choices, one meal at a time.

To help you see that you can afford to make a better choice, I want to show you the breakdown of what fresh and frozen fruits and veggies cost compared to a child's fast-food meal.

- *A five-pound bag of frozen carrots and peas costs $4.17. That means you can make twenty-five dinners, serving your child 2/3 cup of veggies each time!*

- *A five-pound bag of rice costs $5.75, so if you serve your child 1/2 cup of rice, the bag will provide around twenty-two dinners.*

- *A five-pound bag of black beans (as a chicken substitute for vegetarians) costs $7.00 and offers up twenty one-half cup servings (cooked).*

- *A 6.5-pound bag of frozen chicken breasts costs $15.00 and offers thirty-four meals of a three-ounce chicken breast.*

- *A five-pound bag of apples is $4.99.*

For only $1.21 a meal, you can have a healthy, well-balanced lunch or dinner of chicken breast, black beans, rice and veggies for your child twenty times a month, with two servings of rice left over and fourteen servings of chicken left over.

A child's fast-food meal costs between $2.99 and $5.99 depending on the time of year and where you live. It offers almost no nutritional value and is high in fat, sodium, sugar and calories.

If you are feeding your child or your whole family fast food several times a week, you are most likely spending between sixty to one hundred fifty dollars a week depending on the size of your family!

I recently did a show on ABC for the Live Well Network's "Deals" on how to stretch your meals to save money. You can buy a whole chicken and make two trays of chicken enchiladas out of five ingredients that will feed your family for a week! (Look for Green Chile Chicken Enchiladas in my recipe section). You can also buy one 3.5 pound chicken for $3.49 on sale, grab a bag of frozen mixed veggies for $7.55 (six-pound bag!) and make a stir-fry as well as have enough chicken left over to make a huge batch of Ethel's Easy Chicken Salad (also in my recipe section) to take to work for the week or send with your kids to school. As a side note, organic or at least natural, hormone and antibiotic-free chicken is always preferable and can be found as cheaply as $4.97 a pound for boneless, skinless breasts (HEB Houston).

These prices show that you *can* get your kids the daily nutrition they need at a price that's not going to break your budget.

Let your children see you budgeting and show them how important it is to you that they eat fresh, well-balanced, home-cooked meals.

Teach your kids to be part of the solution, not part of the problem.

FACT:
Research shows that obese children are more than three times as likely to be hospitalized as those who are not obese.[4]

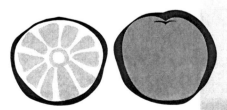

Annual medical costs for a child diagnosed with obesity are on average three times higher than those for a child who is not overweight or obese.

Nationwide, it is estimated that annual costs for prescription drugs, emergency room treatment and outpatient services related to childhood obesity total more than $14 billion, with an additional $238 million in inpatient hospital costs.[5]

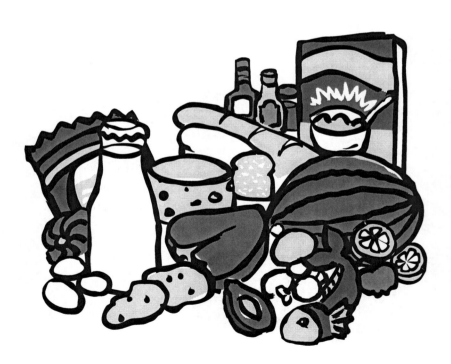

Break the Sugar Cycle

I feel powerless and sometimes angry at the amount of junk food our kids are exposed to each day. Most of that junk food contains some form of real or fake sugar: high fructose corn syrup, aspartame (NutraSweet), saccharin (Sweet 'n Low) or sucralose (Splenda). All of these sugar substitutes are considered toxic by many and are dangerous choices for both children and adults.[6] Considering how often our kids are exposed to them in junk food, sodas and sugary cereals, we need to sit up and pay attention. Often the moment our kids leave the house, the sugar cycle begins for them.

Possibly they had chocolate milk, orange juice and or a dessert for lunch at school—moms, this is *a lot* of sugar for their little brains and bodies! Then maybe they answered the most questions correctly in music class, so they got some Skittles as a reward. Then, a classmate had a birthday and the mom brought donut holes for everyone, so they had several of those on the playground for recess. After school, a kind grandparent or baby sitter, or the after-school program, gives them frozen yogurt with Oreos on top. Finally, after their softball, soccer or baseball practice in the evening, usually before dinner, a well-intentioned but poorly educated—when it comes to food—mom has brought Rice Krispy treats and a red sports drink for a snack. Now it's time for dinner. If you go eat out, the cycle continues with salty, starchy kids' food and dessert and probably nothing green on their plate.

If you make the wise choice to eat at home, is your child going to want a fabulously healthy dinner, where he can actually taste the true flavors of the multiple steamed or roasted veggies he's getting, the grilled chicken and brown rice or quinoa? No way! It's going to taste like bland cardboard to him after all the super sweet and salty things he has eaten all day. That's what makes it so difficult for moms to get our kids to eat "real", whole, clean food at dinner.

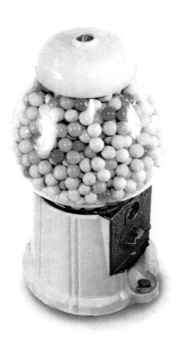

FACT:
The financial cost of child-hood obesity tips the scales at $3 billion annually.[8]

SUGAR: WHY IT'S NOT SO SWEET

We've already mentioned that kids in the United States consume 300 or more calories a day from sugar-containing beverages . . . but what about from other sources? US teens consume an overall **four pounds** of sugar a week.[7]

According to Nancy Appleton, PhD, author of **Lick the Sugar Habit** and Dr. Kathleen DesMaisons, author of **Little Sugar Addicts**, here are just a few ways sugar can ruin your health:

- **Sugar acts like a drug in the body and affects the same brain chemicals that heroin and morphine do.** (DesMaisons)

- **The biochemistry of sugar sensitivity is an underlying factor in alcoholism, addiction, depression, ADD, obesity and diabetes.** (DesMaisons)

- **Sugar can cause a rapid rise of adrenaline, hyperactivity, anxiety, difficulty concentrating and crankiness in children.** (Appleton)

- **Sugar feeds cancer cells and has been connected to the development of cancer.** (Appleton)

- **Sugar contributes to obesity.** (Appleton)

Step by Step: Take Ownership

Break your family's junk-food cycle by making a better choice for your child and yourself! Some of us have a family history of obesity, being overweight and many of the illnesses associated with excess weight. Do something about it now. Be the catalyst for change in your home and with your family. It begins with a simple step. Don't default to "Obesity runs in my family" or "We're all just built this way." More and more research is showing that obesity is *not* genetic, but a result of lifestyle choices. To quote Judith Stern of the University of California, Davis, "Genetics load the gun and (diet) environment pulls the trigger." We tend to fall back on what we know as "normal" and excuse unhealthy eating behaviors. We then say that the reason a child looks a certain way is that it's genetic, when in reality it a result of habits in the home that have carried on for generations. Don't give your kids an out or an excuse. Make a decision to change the next generation in your family so they can teach their kids and grandkids as well. I have clients and friends who say that they have always been heavy so there is no hope for their child and they actually tell their child that, giving the younger generation an excuse to eat poorly. They rationalize by saying they are making their children feel better when in reality they are setting them up to fail and fall back into the same patterns that have been happening generation after generation because of what they are seeing being modeled in their own home.

No one is going to do the work for you. Make a decision that if your kids turn out a certain way you can at least take personal responsibility and have an active role in the outcome. Take the offensive. Don't be a passive observer in your child's health and life and just hope for the best.

I know many of you are concerned about the cost associated with buying "organic or natural" products but in reality, wellness is less expensive than treating illness, and 99 percent of all disease comes from what goes into our bodies—frequent doctor visits add up. Prevention is the best cure! Take it one step at a time, start integrating more whole, natural, "real" foods into your kids' diets—and your own! —and then sit back and watch how things change. You might be pleasantly surprised.

Kids who consider themselves overweight are

- two times as likely to consider themselves not smart enough;

- three times as likely to worry about their futures;

- four times as likely to have poor family relationships; and five times as likely to have low self-esteem.[9]

Establish Structure

When it comes to healthy eating, it's important to start from an early age by establishing routine, structure, rules and roles—and to plan ahead. Otherwise, you will quickly discover that the little ones have taken over and they are running the show. That's when mom and dad start to get wiped out and behavior starts to go down the tubes—both the parents' and the kids'. This can start at a very young age, so people, you've got to have a plan. Don't play defense, play offense. Discipline, rule following and boundary setting are a very important part of your child's emotional and intellectual growth. Without them your home and the world in general would be in chaos. Today, I am seeing fewer and fewer parents with the desire or energy to stand up to their kids and set rules and boundaries. As a result, I see more and more aggressive, confused, unhealthy and unhappy kids. Kids need to be led, and as a parent that's your job, in every area of their lives.

We have a framed photo in a special place in our home that outlines the "Laws" of our home. We created these laws together as a family when the kids were younger and they are very simple and easy to understand. The frame is in a location where everyone can see it daily, and it's printed clearly, in a nice big, red font. That way, when my children do something that goes against the Laws of our house and I have to choose a consequence for them, I don't have to get angry—although Lord knows I'm not perfect and do get emotional every now and then—we can calmly refer back together to the Laws and the kids understand that they have disobeyed without me having to repeat myself over and over again.

Here's what it looks like:

Laws of Our House

Ask

Obey

Forgive

Share

Respect

Be kind

Be truthful

Once you have established the Laws of your home, when a child refuses to follow them, rather than scream yell or throw a fit—as a child would—simply smile and say, "I'm sorry you don't want to eat your green beans, but one of the laws of our house is to obey." Then you continue the conversation you were having with your husband or another child. It's hard for a child to argue when he tries to draw you in and you constantly say, with a smile on your face, "I love you too much to argue" and continue your other conversation. It takes the winds right out of their sails. Maybe not the first time, but if you are consistent, they realize they have nowhere to go, and they must comply; it defuses their emotion. Who wants to sit through a dinner night after night where one or more kids refuse to eat anything or any vegetables? Your fun family time at the table becomes a nightmare. Sticking to the laws allows you to cut it off before you are thirty minutes into the meal and everyone is miserable.

There are ten rules that we like to follow in our home and that I recommend to my clients to keep them on track. They're simple to follow and easy to remember.

Ten Rules of Healthy Family Eating

1. Practice the "Our Family" way of eating

Make it clear to your kids that this is how "Our Family" eats. Just make sure you're eating it too, or you will lose all credibility! Kids look to their parents first, then to their older siblings to set an example. If you don't practice what you preach with them, you've lost before you even started. This is especially true when it comes to choosing "real" food over fast food, choosing water over soft drinks—"liquid candy"—and making home-cooked meals and exercising on a regular basis.

2. Limit Options

Despite what restaurants and the media try to convince us of by making special menus for kids, there should be no difference between kids' food and our food, unless we parents prefer highly spiced food or the child has certain allergies or food intolerances that prevent them from eating certain food groups. This may sound harsh at first, but when you take out the negotiation, the power shifts back to you and it teaches them that they should be eating the same food that you are whether you are at home or eating out. Think about what things were like before the advent of fast food and drive-ins in the '60s. Everyone ate the same thing! Whatever mom put on the table, that's what you got. I know this might sound like it goes against the current trend of "giving your kids choices" to foster independence, but it really doesn't. You can still give them choices, but you choose which vegetables get to be part of their selection.

3. Don't Give Up

Statistically, children have to try something fifteen times before their palette accepts it. If you give up the first time, you've lost. Be consistent and persistent and don't give up! Use the "Our Family" motto: say "This is what Our Family is eating tonight," and smile a big genuine smile. Even if they only take a few bites, you are on the road to success.

4. Skip "Fun" Food

Don't buy any packaged cereal or snack labeled as "Fun" and don't buy foods just because they are "vitamin enriched." Stick to the periphery of the grocery store and don't set foot in the center aisles.[10] Don't let your kids pick the groceries that go in the cart if they are making bad choices. Who's paying for the groceries? You or them? If it's too hard to make good choices with your kids at the store, find a way to leave them at home or with a friend.

5. Take the Generation Test

Start giving your kids "real" food, not processed food in a bag or wrapper that's full of preservatives, pesticides, artificial coloring and genetically modified ingredients. If there are more than five to seven ingredients or something your grandmother or anyone from an older generation wouldn't recognize on the label, don't buy it.

6. Create Some Wiggle Room

Come up with your own set of rules and compromises that work for you and your family, like the 90/10 or even 80/20 rule where you eat well 80 percent of the time and the other 20 percent you just don't worry about it. But if you have to make a bad choice, make a "better" bad choice. Try to choose treats or options that are still healthy. If you do this from a young age, your kids won't even realize you are doing it. Once they are older, teach them how to make the better choice themselves by pointing out options at both the grocery and restaurants. Berries with cream or a huge piece of chocolate cake? Several dark chocolate squares or a fudge pop?

7. Practice Portion Awareness

Our kids are growing larger and larger as a result of the "Supersize Me" mentality. As portions have increased in size over the past fifteen years, so have we. Parents, hear me now: Less is

More! Serve your child a plate appropriate for them and don't eat family style. It encourages overeating and it's hard to keep track of how much you have eaten. A friend with three kids recently shared that her mother brought them up eating their dinner on salad plates. While this idea might not work for a thirteen-year-old boy who is growing rapidly and needs more calories, it's a good idea overall. Even discouraging your child from seconds is appropriate if you are serving them an adequate amount of food for their age. Know your child and pay attention to what they are eating so that you are able to make good serving decisions for them at home.

Twenty years ago, the average soda serving was six-and-a-half ounces and eighty-five calories. Today it's about twenty ounces and three hundred calories. We don't need this excess and neither do our kids. Consuming an extra hundred calories a day for a year without burning them up can lead to a weight gain of ten pounds per year. That could be a life-threatening number for a young child.

Once again, you need to model portion awareness for your kids as well. Don't go to the movies and order the largest popcorn and soda. If you decide to treat yourself, order the smallest size and then split that with your child. At home, make sure snacks are individually wrapped or prepared; no eating out of the box or walking around the house with food. Sit at the table and serve your kids a preprepared serving to ensure healthy serving sizes. You can save money as well by buying snacks in bulk, like pretzels, and then individually putting them into snack bags that suit your child's age and food needs. Finally, I like to serve my kids their dinner on a large salad plate. The adult-size dinner plates hold too much food, even for adults. Give them portions that are appropriate for their size: they can always come back for more.

Healthy Example: apples with peanut butter, or homemade trail mix. Hummus and baby carrots, sesame sticks, watermelon.

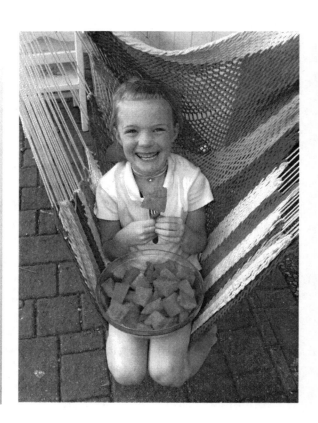

8. Teach Food Quality

I was recently speaking at a local elementary school and pointed out to a mom that if a child's only exposure to veggies is the under-ripe tomato slice and limp lettuce on a fast-food burger, can you blame her for disliking vegetables? Good food quality leads to good food flavor. Point out the differences to your child and try to only make quality choices both in what you buy and where you choose to eat out—i.e., no fast food.

9. Don't Be Afraid to Say "NO"

This is a big one. The entitlement we see in kids these days is staggering. When did they become the boss? If you're the one paying for and cooking the food, and they are still living under your roof, you get to make the choices. Period. Parents are now taking a backseat to their kids' wants and desires and look where it's gotten us as a nation. If our children were capable of making these good decisions themselves, they wouldn't live at home until they are eighteen. Once again, if there are only good choices in the house, they will only be able to make a good choice. Remove temptation for both you and your kids. If you know you love a certain unhealthy snack food and will end up eating a whole bag or box, don't buy it. If you know your children love a certain un-healthy cookie and you aren't able to be home to monitor what they're eating, don't buy it. Set yourself up for success, not failure. Finally, don't succumb to the badgering. Kids are tenacious, so you need to teach them early on that "no" means "no" and "What I say, You obey."

10. Don't be Afraid to Talk to Kids about the Effects of Food on Their Bodies

The number of overweight people in the world, 1.1 billion, now equals the number of undernourished people. Houston, we have a problem. Some parents feel if they bring up the topic of weight or appearance or comment on their child's food choices, it will negatively affect their child's ego in some way, so they choose to say nothing and stand by, watching their kids become heavier and sicker day by day. Then, once the child reaches a point where the doctor says their health is at risk, the parents are obligated to step in and make some radical changes. Don't fall for that. Talk to your kids. Explain to them what's happening to people in our country and why, and that it's your job to teach and protect them while they are still in your home. It's much easier to be proactive than to go back at age ten and have to police and patrol everything that goes in their mouths because they have become obese and are at risk for serious, life-threatening diseases. It's also cheaper!

Routine

Regardless of the type of personality your child ends up exhibiting, no one comes out of the womb already structured and ready to conquer the world. They don't come out asking for a certain napping or feeding schedule—wouldn't that be nice? As parents we have to figure it out ourselves; sometimes with the help of a spouse, family member or other caregiver, and sometimes alone. We, as parents, set structure and routine from the day they are born: we decide what time to feed them, change them when they are dirty and put them down for naps or put them down at night to sleep. Do we let them cry a little, not at all or until they fall asleep? These are our choices to make. Whatever plan we decide on, routine provides safety, boundaries and security for our children.

FACT:
A kids' meal cheeseburger, small fry and small soda packs an unbelievable 635 calories!

Don't wait until all heck has broken lose at home. Set some guidelines in place early on that you think work for you as a family, and stick to them. Granted, as children grow, you must be fluid and adapt your guidelines to their changing needs, but establish a routine for your home that is basically set. Repeat the rules over and over to your kids and yourself.

In many ways, you must run your family as you would run a business. Do you want it to fall apart? Go bankrupt emotionally or financially? If the kids are running the house, you can bet you will be well on your way to the demise of the corporation. Give them an inch, they take a mile. "Why can't I just have one more dessert, mom, it's a healthy one: flavored yogurt?" Then you think, "oh, they need their calcium" to justify the fact that you don't want to argue, so you give in and a few years down the road, you realize your child has been loading up on two "healthy desserts" every night, and now they have a weight issue, a health issue and are being made fun of by their friends.

A great way to keep this problem from happening is to focus on establishing a family routine, even if you can only make it possible a few days out of the week. This will reduce stress for both you and your family around mealtimes because everyone will know what to expect. This also will change with the ages of the children over time, but set a night once a week for you to meet with your spouse or sit by yourself and go over what's working or what's not.

Five Steps to Establishing Routine

1. Preplan Menus

Take time on Sunday night to preplan menus for the evenings you know you will be home. Just because you can't all sit down at the same time as a family every night doesn't means you need to resort to drive-thru or pizza; you can still feed your kids a healthy meal, the *same* meal, separately at different times.

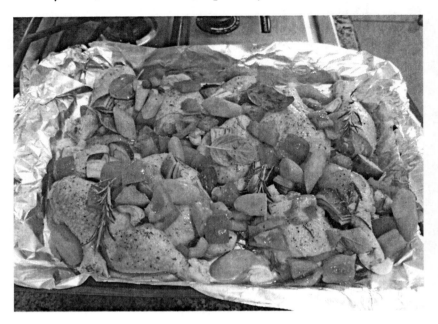

2. Eat as a Family Whenever Possible

Why are we no longer eating for pleasure over a long meal together, for family connection and for community? The process of eating and sharing a meal together is much more than putting food into our bodies. "If it were just about food, we would squirt it into their mouths with a tube," says Robin Fox, an anthropologist who teaches at Rutgers University in New Jersey, about the mysterious way that family dinner engraves our souls. "A meal is about civilizing children. It's about teaching them to be a member of their culture."[11]

Why have some of us broken it down scientifically into getting the "nutrients" or sustenance we need for the day, even if they are being consumed while driving around in the car? Historically, sharing a meal together represented a bonding experience between family and friends and a coming together of community.

Statistics show that families—and that includes families with both one and two parents—who sit down together at least four nights a week have closer and more open relationships with their kids. And that means dining with no TV, no computers and no cell phones—no screens at all! That goes for you, too, Mom. Mealtime may be when you will learn the most about your kids. Mine never cease to surprise me with some new piece of information at dinner, either about themselves or a friend. Just like any other relationship, spending time together is key for nurturing your connection with your children, and eating together is a great daily activity you can do as a family.

Studies show that the more often families eat together, the less likely kids are to smoke, drink, do drugs, get depressed, develop eating disorders and consider suicide, and the more likely they are to do well in school, delay having sex, eat their vegetables, learn big words and know which fork to use.[12]

3. Dine at Home

Don't be a stranger to your kitchen; most of America has forgotten where the kitchen is! Try to eat at home as much as possible and make your kitchen the heart of the home again. That way you can also control the quality and the quantity of the food your kids are eating. Make good substitutes and teach them how to upgrade their choices, like choosing brown rice over pasta or lean chicken over fatty red meat.

4. Avoid Kids' Menus When Eating Out

Most of the time kids' menus are not made up of "real" food. The options are primarily fried and the food is often completely devoid of nutrients. Instead, order from the regular menu for both you and your child, or if the child is very young, bring food from home. If you have to go out, make good choices for your waistline and your wallet, like splitting an entrée with your child or have them split one with each other. Avoid family-style restaurants, which can lead to overeating and always order something green for your child on the side. I am known for taking a container of sliced bell peppers and steamed broccoli with me on the nights we have multiple sports games and I know we are going to be eating out somewhere where vegetables and/or fruit are not offered.

5. Eat Dessert on Your Own Turf

We know that we are always better off when we control the quality and quantity of food our kids are eating. This especially applies to desserts, where the sugar content is bound to be higher. Recent studies are showing that sugar may lead to cancer.[13]

Since kids now believe that they should get a dessert every night and at school lunch, and they are getting so many sweets outside of the home at friends' houses, birthday parties and sporting events, we have to step in and control their sugar intake when we can. Tell your children before you go to the restaurant, movies or ball field that they are going to have better dessert options at home. Let them pick out some healthy dessert choices at the store so they know what's waiting for them at home. Planning in advance will help avoid any conflict once you arrive at your location and, once again, you will be saving money along with taking care of your kids' health.

SOME OF MY KIDS' FAVORITE HEALTHY DESSERTS

- Dark chocolate squares
- Dreyer's Whole Fruit Popsicles
- Sorbet of any kind
- Mini ice-cream sandwiches
- Stonyfield Farms Chocolate Frozen Yogurt Pops
- All-natural "GoodPop" frozen pops
- Fresh mixed berries
- Frozen grapes or tangerines
- Strawberries dipped in Greek yogurt and frozen

Eating Right: It Takes a Village

Today, we have every imaginable combination of people caring for our kids: parents who are married, single, divorced, grandparents who live in, grandparents who watch kids while we are at work, day-care employees, nannies and housekeepers. Each one of these individuals has a role in the raising of our child and it almost always involves food. Ensuring that everyone is on the same page when it comes to food is *the* key to successful healthy eating at home. For example, if you want your children to eat only organic food, you not only need to provide that food if you are away at work, but you must also explain to the caregiver that it is not acceptable to take your eighteen-month-old out for a late afternoon snack of soda and fries.

It's critical to have these conversations up front to avoid any conflict or miscommunication, and make sure you check in weekly to make sure things are going well. Caregivers often see themselves as a "grandparent" type and will tend to indulge the kids on an ongoing basis. Set ground rules and stick with them: you know what's right for your child.

Capitalizing on Different Parenting Styles

Moms and dads, just like men and women, do things differently. Period. You are rarely going to do things the exact same way as your spouse, so let it go unless it's something that could be harmful to your child. Unless you see your child suffering mentally, emotionally or physically, agree to disagree on some issues, but make sure you are not sabotaging the other's efforts. This was very common in my home for the first two kids: I would get so mad that my husband couldn't remember the "schedule" for food or naps or the right way to burp or swaddle. I mean really, how hard could it be? Well, it was hard for him. He wasn't there all the time, he was working and many men just aren't wired that way, even if you write it down. It's essential to learn to accept what your significant other can and can't do, and just move on. Work together as a sports team would; use your strengths and differences to your advantage. In the end, your kids will benefit from both styles.

Play up each other's natural strengths and preferences. Is one of you a late night owl and the other an early riser? Take advantage of that and develop a system with your children and their meals that keeps both of you from being run down and taking the easy way out.

Does one of you have more job flexibility than the other or is one of you a much better cook? Choose that person to be in charge of the weekly schedule or meal planning for the family, so it's not left to last minute decisions all the time, which usually end up being junk food or Pizza Trap nights. The most important thing is to keep everyone in the loop about the kids' schedule, eating and otherwise, so that there is consistency in your children's lives. I finally got this through my thick skull and realized that I couldn't always be at home, so I printed out a copy of our daughters' schedules to put on the fridge so whoever was with our daughters would know what to do. I also learned that my way wasn't the only way and that my kids would survive if someone deviated from the schedule. This, my friend, was a tough lesson.

Use Older Siblings to Support Your Cause

This takes us back to the "it's ok to be sneaky" mentality. Sometimes we need the older ones to help out, just for the sheer sake of another set of hands—and they should be expected to help. At the same time, the younger ones will look to see what and how their older siblings are eating. Bring the older siblings on board. If they are already making good choices, this will be easier. If they aren't, well then it's time to start!

Do your older kids, over the age of five, sit at the table, engage in conversation—well, maybe at least some conversation, depending on whether you have a teenager—and eat a reasonable dinner? If not, you have a problem. These are all reasonable expectations for a child of that age and older. Most are expected to do it at school in the cafeteria, so why not at home?

Tweens and teens are very interested in the way they look and the way they perform in sports. If they understand that eating healthily will help their complexion, their hair and nails, or make them stronger for athletics, they will pay more attention to what they are eating. Hopefully they will eliminate the junk when they associate it with acne, poor energy, inability to concentrate and mood swings—not to mention their waistlines. Younger siblings will notice this and ask questions. Hopefully, they will want to follow suit.

For instance, when a high school student living off junk food hears that Stanford just spent $23.9 million dollars on a new college dining hall that offers carefully selected combinations of local, seasonal, organic and natural foods to help athletes meet performance targets, learn about wellness and recover from illness or sports related injuries, they become a lot more interested in food and what it can do for them.[14]

Use this to your advantage; keep your tweens and teens up to speed on new healthy food research—not fads or diets—and present the findings to them in a way that is easily relatable. If they are into athletics, show them all the information online about how many NBA and NFL teams are hiring personal chefs to help their players perform better, deal with gluten and dairy intolerances, lengthen the duration of their careers, recover more rapidly from injury and just feel better in general.

"*Watch your thoughts,*
they become your words,
watch your words,
they become your actions.
Watch your actions,
they become your habits,
watch your habits,
they become your character.
Watch your character,
it becomes your destiny."

—AUTHOR UNKNOWN

ACNE AND JUNK FOOD

Want a simple, inexpensive and pain-free way to clear up your skin? Clean up your diet!

A Poor Diet Is Bad for Your Skin
—Dr. Mark Hyman, MD[15]

- Skin health, and acne in particular, are tied strongly to diet.

- Acne is caused by inflammation and oxidative stress.

- Traditional indigenous cultures have little acne, but as soon as they adopt a Western diet or SAD (Standard American Diet), they see increasing levels of acne.

- Sugar raises insulin levels, which promotes the production of testosterone in women, and inflammation in general, causing acne.

- Saturated and processed fats increase arachidonic acid levels and compete with omega-3 fats in the body, leading to more inflammation and acne.

- Milk and dairy consumption is closely linked with acne (and many other skin and health problems) in part because of the hormones (including growth hormone) in dairy and because of the saturated fats.

- High-sugar milk chocolate can increase acne by increasing inflammation, but dark chocolate does the opposite.

Be Consistent

Consistency is a key factor in maintaining a healthy home environment and also in getting the behavioral results you want from your kids. Consistency, by definition, means that rules and expectations are the same on a daily basis. Consistency means your child knows what to expect from one day to the next and this makes your child's world predictable and less confusing; this also helps them to develop a sense of responsibility. For those of you who have worriers, this enables them to quit worrying about what might happen and also teaches them accountability for their actions.

Children who have consistent rules with predictable consequences are less likely to "push the limits" and constantly test their parents by misbehaving. They learn quickly that "no" means "no." Investing early in consistent parenting will pay off in the future. There will be fewer temper tantrums as your child grows older, and significantly less arguing and bargaining for what they want. Remember the pester and persistence factors at the grocery store? If you consistently respond in the same way each time from a very early age, your child will learn that nagging will get them nowhere.

Consistency in the home and around mealtime structure also helps in the parent/child bonding process and will eventually lead to less chaos around mealtime as the child grows older.

Consistency is challenging for parents because in our busy world where moms are tired and spread thin, it's very tempting to give in and to let children do whatever they want. As moms, we become tired and sometimes doubt our own judgment. We start to think "Am I being too hard on them? They're just kids. Maybe I should back down." This is not the answer.

When their lives are consistent, children will gain the self-confidence they need to grow and become more and more confident and independent, which makes your life easier overall. Have faith in yourself and continue to persevere; it will pay off in the long run.

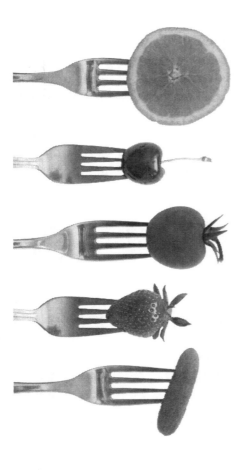

FACT:
As of 2010,
6.7 % of kids
under age five
are overweight
or obese[16]

Empathy Works

What is empathy, exactly? According to Merriam-Webster, empathy is "being aware of and sharing another person's feelings, experiences, and emotions." To be empathetic, you must be aware of your own feelings as well as your child's. This will enable you to be sympathetic to their needs, and to treat them as you expect others outside your home to treat them. Understanding the feelings behind their actions will also help you better cope with their behavior in the tween and teen years. Does this mean you have to be a pushover? No! It just means you can't ignore their feelings, which almost always dictate their behavior. Remember, if your child is acting out, try to look for the feeling or emotion behind the behavior.

To raise a healthy, happy child and to get the appropriate behavior we want out of our kids, without a lot of struggle—we hope—we must appear to be genuinely empathetic when they resist. However, we must also persist when they resist, in a non-confrontational way.

And believe me, if you don't start on this route early and stick to your guns, they will resist. At a very young age, children, as well as their parents, learn to use food as a bargaining chip. Even parents who have always fed their kids the "right way" may encounter an experience with a surprisingly stubborn child.

Having an empathetic attitude towards your kids when they are resistant toward change is the key to getting the results you want from them, whether you're trying to get them to experience a new food or clean their room. Being empathetic works from the day you bring them home from the hospital until the day they leave for college.

No one likes—or responds well to—a dictator or an authoritarian person. Saying "You will eat your broccoli or I will make you!" won't get you far. When you choose to run your home that way, or respond to kids' feelings that way, more often than not you are going to be met with resistance, hatred or passive-aggressive behavior. Does this get you the end result you want? Maybe, but your child never really learns the correct behavior or does it on his own—he's doing it because he has to.

Show some empathy. In a kind and caring voice, use phrases like, "I'm so sorry you feel that way," or enforceable statements like "We will eat as soon as you are seated," or "Breakfast is served for the next fifteen minutes. Get what you need to hold you until lunch." When your children push back at the dinner table, show them that you feel and understand their emotions. But also make the boundaries clear—don't budge from them.

For more tips on enforceable statements and how to use empathy with your kids, visit LoveandLogic.com, a teaching website for parents and educators.

FACT:
As your weight goes up, the size and function
of your brain goes down.
—Dr. Daniel Amen, www.amenclinics.com

Persistence Pays Off

Accept the idea that you are in this for the long haul. Try not to become emotional or get upset over your children's stubbornness. Keep smiling and keep serving the good stuff. Let them know that your will is like iron.

There will be days when you think it's not worth it and want to give in, but remember, parenting is a marathon, not a sprint. You can do it! Set yourself up for success by setting easy goals for your family that can be achieved daily. If you look too far ahead, you may feel overwhelmed. Children look for stability in their parents. Even though they continually test the boundaries, it brings them peace and comfort. You need to be more persistent than they are; don't back down. Eventually, good eating becomes a habit and then it becomes part of your family's lifestyle. Stick with it and you will experience less and less resistance.

When my youngest daughter Gigi started eating "real" food—not out of a baby jar!—I was determined to get her eating like the others, with a well-balanced meal for both lunch and dinner. So each night, I put one baby organic carrot on her plate and one green bean along with everything else. No matter what, I was determined to keep putting the vegetables on her plate even though she refused them every night. Everyone would laugh at me and say "She is too young and she is so stubborn, she is never going to eat them!" I knew that at some point, she would just decide to eat it, and I was right! One night, I looked over and she had picked the carrot up in her cute little one-and-a-half-year-old hands, looked at her sisters eating theirs, looked at me and took a big bite with a huge smile on her face. It was one of the happiest moments for me because my persistence paid off. (As a side note, now she is six and very dramatic and we still struggle sometimes at night with certain new foods and textures, but I haven't given up!)

Be empathetic, but persistent. Telling your children "I love you too much to argue"—one of my favorite one-liners from LoveandLogic.com—with a genuine smile on your face, works well when dealing with resistance. But it must be genuine or it won't work! I have been using this technique now for eleven years and it works just as well with an eleven-year-old as it does with a three-year-old, which fascinates me.

You're the parent and you must know and believe that you are making the right choice for your kids in the long run. Don't give in. If you don't teach your children how to make the choices that will keep them healthy for life, who will? It's your responsibility to fight for them and their health in an eating culture that makes it very difficult for them to do it for themselves.

Say "No" to Negotiation

Negotiation can work well when it's between two adult equals. When you throw a child in the mix, it's a recipe for disaster.

In some homes, one of the parents is going to refuse to comply. I see this over and over again with clients, where the mom says, "My husband likes his junk food and soft drinks and chips. It makes it really hard for me to make changes in the house because the kids ask why Daddy doesn't have to do it." Or to hear it from the kids, "Daddy doesn't like vegetables and neither do I." This is a great teachable moment with kids. You can explain to them that we—mom and kids or dad and kids—are doing our own new thing, which is nonnegotiable, or "I love you too much to argue." And that daddy—or mommy—is a grown-up who can decide for himself what he chooses to put into his body. But say it with empathy; never disparage the person who is not yet on board with the new eating habits of your house. Don't make the other adult in the house look bad in your children's eyes, just explain that when they are adults, they will be able to make their own decisions as well.

SAY GOOD-BYE TO HUMILIATING PUBLIC FREAK OUTS

When you go to the mall, and your three-year-old wants a big gulp soda from the closest place in the food court or a big piece of candy, instead of buying it to temporarily appease them, don't be afraid to smile and say "No, not today honey." When they pitch a fit, you just keep smiling and say "I love you too much to argue." Yes, everyone around you might be glaring and staring, but you must know as a mother that you are doing the right thing for your child in the long run. You are setting boundaries early and keeping them healthy. You are the boss! They might continue to scream the first few times, but after that, you will begin to notice that the duration is shorter and eventually they just quit asking all together.

I have had many clients say to me, "I am so worried because my child's not eating anything, if he just eats something at dinner or lunch I'll be happy." So what does he end up eating? Exactly what he wants: junk. And so the pattern is set. Are we that resigned and unwilling to set higher standards for our kids, where "just eating anything" is enough? Has it become that bad?

When our kids are babies, we nurse them or give them high quality formula, and then slowly begin to add in healthy fruits, whole grains and vegetables. We closely monitor the amounts, their reaction for a possible allergy, how often they eat, and if they are growing as they should be each time we visit the doctor. How did we transform from that caring, involved, sometimes overly protective mother monitoring our child's diet so closely to accepting him putting anything into his mouth?

Instant gratification is not what your child needs to be healthy or happy, even though in the short run it might seem to calm things down in the car, at the mall or around the house. But you know what happens to children who get everything they want? They keep asking for more.

You're the parent and you must know and believe that you are making the right choice for your kids in the long run. Don't give in. If you don't teach them how to make the choices that will keep them healthy for life, who will?

When my family and I eat out, our kids share an adult entrée of something healthy or I always order a side of steamed broccoli or green beans and substitute fruit for fries if they get a kids' order. It's a habit now for us and they expect it; in fact, they usually order it themselves. They know the importance of having a rainbow plate and have learned over time that they actually feel better when they eat this way.

Remember persistence and resistance? Teach and be strong. You are the boss.

Don't be afraid to tell your kids "no" when the ice cream truck pulls up after soccer or baseball and they haven't had dinner yet: be firm! Go back to the "I love you too much to argue." (LoveandLogic.com)

Stand Up for Healthy Eating

Parents, you can't be a nutritional pushover. Don't be afraid to stand up for your child and ask for better options, wherever you are!

Are you tired of what's being sold at the concession stand during sports games at your school? In your school cafeteria? In the fellowship hall at church? At the food court in the mall? At the movies? Junk food is everywhere. You have to take a stand and have a voice if you want to make a change and be heard. By doing so, you'll teach your kids eventually to do the same and stand up for themselves and their own health.

If you don't like the food at your child's school or day care, say something. I often speak at local elementary schools and love watching how the moms come together to accomplish change within the school community. At a recent lecture, I was given a tour of the school's new organic garden that two mothers had planted, along with the help of the children. By taking a chance, asking for what they wanted and following up with a lot of hard work, these two mothers have permanently impacted the lives of thousands of students for years to come.

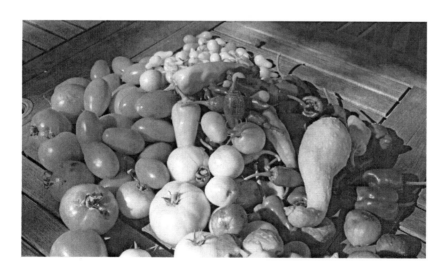

MOM'S TIPS FOR SPEAKING UP FOR YOUR KIDS: HOW YOU CAN MAKE A DIFFERENCE IN YOUR CHILD'S WORLD

1. Start a mom's group at school. You are probably already familiar with the parents who are like-minded when it comes to what the kids are eating. Don't be afraid to reach out to them and set up a bimonthly or weekly time to talk and share ideas. There is power and influence in numbers. Jot down a list of ideas and positive suggestions for the person who controls the food where your kids go to school or day care and give it to officials who can make a difference. Offer to help plan meals or to consult on a regular basis with whoever handles food service.

2. Put together a positive e-mail, letter or petition stating your concerns and the changes you would like made. You can even send it to your local newspaper. I see

more and more editorials on our nation's children and health and many moms writing letters to the editor expressing their concerns.

3. At your child's school or day care, bring in a public speaker to talk to the moms, teachers and kids about nutrition and making good food choices. Educating parents as well as children and staff will start to move everyone toward the same goal.

4. Arrange for a local speaker to speak to a smaller group of children privately in someone's home, church or community center—you can even do this through Girl Scouts or Boy Scouts of America. I am the troop leader for my daughter's Girl Scout troop and we have spoken to the girls several years in a row about nutrition and the importance of eating healthy food, or "grow food." Look for people you know in your community who would be willing to help out and don't be afraid to ask them to speak to your kids!

Accentuate the Positive: Praise Goes Far

Praise is a very powerful tool in getting the results you want from your child, whether it's picking up her room, getting better grades in school or trying a new vegetable that's on her plate without being asked.

When my kids were very young, I learned from my daughters' music teacher the positive results of pointing out in front of others, or noticing "out loud" when a child is following directions or doing what you asked. Instead of pointing out which child was not following directions, she praised the child who was doing what she asked. Magically, all of the other four-year-olds looked over at the child who was being praised and copied that child's behavior. Children love it when you brag about them in front of others. It's important to praise them when they are obeying, not just criticize when they disobey, and as parents sometimes we forget that, especially when we have three or four children. This is especially true around the hectic mealtime hour where we more often than not feel frazzled.

When you praise and recognize your child's behavior out loud, especially in front of others, you are giving the best in positive reinforcement. Use praise at mealtimes around the dinner table as a means of acknowledging your child's bravery and positive attitude when it comes to trying new foods. Brag about them in front of their siblings.

What does this praise sound like?

"I love how Brian already has his napkin in his lap." I use this one a lot when all of the others are eating and have forgotten to put their napkins in the proper place.

"I love how Elizabeth is eating all of her carrots without being asked." This one works well when the others *aren't* eating their carrots.

This will encourage *all* your children to be adventurous and try new foods because they know they'll receive your praise.

When are YOU as a parent going to take responsibility for your child's health?

"A child's education begins with educating the parents."

—ROBERT DOMAN JUNIOR, FOUNDER/DIRECTOR, THE NATIONAL ASSOCIATION FOR CHILD DEVELOPMENT

ACKNOWLEDGE HEALTHY ACTIONS

Congratulate your children and reward them with a nonedible reward every time they fill up a complete color wheel—through their diet—with all the colors of the rainbow. You can do this by keeping a dry erase board in the kitchen. Draw the wheel and let your kids fill it in each time they eat a different colored fruit or veggie.

Pin up the menu from your school's cafeteria so you can talk together the night before about what their options are, and plan how you can make up for whatever unhealthy items they eat with their after school snack and dinner. This way, you make sure they are getting the nutrients they need. For smaller kids, when they get home from school, ask how lunch was so you can determine what kinds of choices they are making. Then you can better reward them for making good choices: a star on a homemade chart tracking the different colored fruits and veggies they eat each day for the little ones, more freedom for older kids like later bedtime on the weekends or a nonedible treat. Star charts go a long way! My ten-year-old is still motivated by receiving stars from her piano teacher.

Let your children put together their own responsibility chart. This is another way to get more help in the kitchen! Make sure to include chef's helper, table setter and clearer, as well as dishwasher as choices for the chart. For younger and possibly more defiant ones, you can include eating their veggies as a responsibility. For the older ones, teaching them to keep track of their own charts is key. Once kids are eating a wide variety of healthy foods, you can start introducing more unique types and flavors of food and track that as well. Once again, you can choose to reward each child in a way that personally motivates him or her.

Check out www.fisher-kids.com. They have put together a very personalized and wonderful responsibility system for children and parents. It's extremely well thought out and allows you to give them praise and other rewards for household chores, including helping out in the kitchen and eating what's on their plate. You can personally customize the system for your family's needs.

Most of all, remember to praise and congratulate your children along the way, even if you encounter a few bumps in the road.

Educate and Empower

You talk to your kids about sex, drugs and alcohol so they are aware and can make better choices. You want them to know what's good for them and what's dangerous. If you want your kids to be "streetwise" about everything that's a potential danger to them it's essential to include food! You have to start early and give them the tools they need to make healthy dietary choices even when you can't be there to make the choice for them.

Our world is so full of distractions, not just for our kids, but for us, too. Any time that we can share our thoughts, dreams and values with our children is beneficial. Even if you are a single parent, you are effecting growth and change in your children's lives by breaking bread and sharing ideas with them. Wouldn't you rather they be influenced by you then by something they watch on TV while eating alone in their room?

We have to stop the cycle of misinformation. Food education is the key to our children's health. It might not be convenient, but it's necessary. Keeping yourself or your kids in the dark is not the answer. Knowledge is power. Children need to understand how food has changed. Most of what we eat now is not nature-made, but man-made and full of synthetic chemicals that can make them sick. They also need to understand how these changes affect their bodies, their performance in school and on the athletic field, and how they feel every day. Unless they know what's really in their food, like HFCS and trans fats, and which foods to avoid to keep those products out of their bodies, how can we expect them to make good choices when we are not around?

Food no longer goes from the ground to our mouths. It has become a huge commercial industry with children as the target. Now is the time to teach your kids about food marketing and how it really works. Children need to understand that food is a business and that they are the clients. I worked to keep my kids away from television for years because I didn't want them exposed to the never-ending cycle of junk-food commercials. I was aware of the influence those commercials would have on their way of thinking. Next time you are shopping with your kids, talk about food marketing and what it is. Point out the sugary cereals and kids' snacks and explain how they are designed to attract kids. Ask them why they think companies would target such unhealthy food to young people.

We were recently eating at a sandwich place and my girls were begging to buy baked chips. My oldest daughter pointed out that the bag said, "All-natural" on the front. I asked her what she thought that meant, and if that really meant they were good for her. After pausing, she turned over the bag and started to read the label. That's my girl! After looking through the ingredients, we soon discovered that many "natural" items can still be bad for you. We have to explain this to our children. Let them know that large, multinational companies will do anything to sell their food. Our kids must know that they can't just read the label and believe it. There are so few marketing restrictions in place when it comes to food that just about anything goes—except in organic labeling.

What really
happens when
our kids hold
the power?

Let Change Be Gradual, But Be 100 Percent Committed

Start slowly, but let your children see that you are 100 percent committed. Make day-by-day changes in the way your family eats. Start evaluating your kids and their needs one by one. Pay attention; who craves what? Does one child prefer salty and sweet snacks while the other prefers loading up on four rolls before dinner? Does one prefer ice cream? Figure out what their triggers are, and make a plan to address them one by one. Look for substitutes. Item by item, clean out your pantry. Get rid of things with more than five to eight ingredients. Get rid of things that are white. Model. Let them see YOU throwing away your diet sodas and carrying around a water bottle. Let them see you change the way you cook at home or the way you eat when you go out. This is not an overnight process. Change takes time, but the time is now. This is a lifestyle change for your family, not a trendy diet you want to follow. Teach them healthy habits, teach them to own them, and they will be theirs for life.

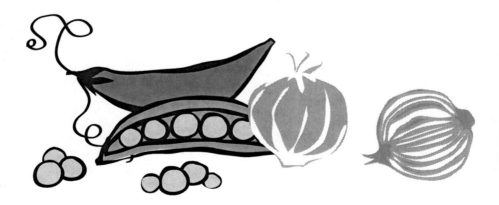

Understand Your Kids

Sure, different kids of different ages have different palettes, as do adults. But how will you know what foods they are drawn to if you don't even try to introduce them to something new? Give them the chance—over time and with your guidance—to discover what they like.

Is your child drawn to all things savory or does she have a sweet tooth? Does she prefer crunchy or soft foods? This is a journey you can take together as you help to shape their palette from a very early age. There are actually scientific reasons why children may be more sensitive to bitter tastes or have a strong sweet tooth. Genes, age, gender and culture all play a big role. That's why each child growing up in the same home can have completely different likes and dislikes when it comes to what they'll eat and what they won't. Your role as a parent is to expose them to as much variety as possible, regardless of what they are naturally drawn to.

Here's how:

- *Always serve a variety of vegetables with each meal; these should encompass half of the meal and will expose them to both bitter and sweet flavors. Sweet: Kids love sweet corn and green peas. Bitter: Braised kale and Swiss chard are full of nutrients and go great with a pot roast and some baked onions and sweet potatoes.*

- *Serve a variety of foods with different textures early on to help overcome any texture issues your child may naturally have. A great way to do this is to serve both raw and cooked veggies. Many kids actually prefer raw, crunchy veggies and by serving them raw you maintain all the nutrients.*

- *Ask questions. If it's not obvious what foods your children are intrinsically drawn to, just ask! They will know what they prefer and why.*

- *Know your child's motivators—Are they money motivated? Do they want more privileges? Do they seek praise?—and use them to your advantage.*

The best way to really understand and get to know your child is around the dinner table. Food naturally gathers people together. How many times have you gone to someone's home for dinner and everyone ends up talking in the kitchen? Where do your kids like to gather when they are at home, especially if they are teens?

Food brings people together and can be a comfort as well. My middle daughter recently said the only time she was homesick at camp was when she sat down to eat each meal. She missed me serving her and missed our family getting together around the dinner table, talking about our day and acting out skits. Time is a precious commodity and so are our kids. Making the effort to get the two together several nights a week is critical.

Studies show that families with the healthiest relationships sit down to dinner together at least four nights a week and actually talk to each other. No screens allowed. If you want an answer to a question that comes up while eating, don't GOOGLE it on your phone or iPad at the table if no one knows the answer. Spend the next twenty minutes talking about what each of you thinks the answer might be and why. It's fun to share ideas. That's when I actually learn the most about my kids. As I said earlier, they never cease to surprise me with some new piece of information at the table.

Back to Basics

We have got to get back to basics, and teach our kids the true value and origin of food. What is an apple? Is it a protein or a carb? What does it do for my body? In what time of year does it grow? If I don't eat apples in the fall, what will my body be missing? Will I get sick more easily?

These are all very important questions that both adults and children should be able to answer about "real" food.

I remember that my own mother became irate when I was in grade school in Texas because the public school district I was in announced that they had discovered a dish that met all of the food group requirements. What was that food? A nacho with fake cheese and salsa and a pickled jalapeno. I thought she was going to lose it. How can any child subsist on nachos—with fake cheese, mind you—for lunch and be a healthy strong child, capable of sitting in a classroom and learning for seven hours a day? Unfortunately, this is still the norm in many schools across the United States today.

Jamie Oliver and his food revolution have done a great job addressing this issue on a national level. His mission to educate people about the adverse effects of sugar and trans fat and junk food in general has literally saved lives all over the world. The knowledge he has given parents and educators on how to retrain their families and students about what to eat or not to eat is remarkable. But is it complicated? No! Jamie is giving people the simplest of facts, even playing show-and-tell in some situations, by emptying a huge dump truck full of sugar in front of parents in California to help people understand how much sugar their kids are eating every year.

DON'T ENCOURAGE YOUR KIDS TO CLEAN THEIR PLATE!

If you are one of those people, like me, who feels compelled to "eat it all," then definitely order a smaller salad plate or appetizer portion. We were all raised to "clean our plate," but the reality is, you don't have to finish what's in front of you if you're full. Teach this to your kids as well. Let them know that it takes twenty minutes for the body to recognize that it's full, and that it's not necessary to be stuffed to be happy. Some kids have a good satiety meter built-in, but most kids are going to need your help.

Make a Game of It

Playing games together at the table is crucial to creating a positive eating experience for young kids. If every meal is a battle, children start to associate negative feelings and pressure with eating and spending time together as a family, which is the last thing you want. If they associate dinner with fun and games, they will look forward to getting together in the evening as a family.

I see this with my children, especially the youngest. When we are all busy and don't share quality time together as a family, they will ask me if we can eat at "the big table" (the big table is the dining room table where we eat as a family). That speaks volumes.

One of the games we like to play goes by several names: roses and thorns, peaks and pits or highs and lows. It's a simple premise where each person goes around the table and shares the high point and low point of their day, week, month, season, etc. It's a great way to connect to what's happening in your children and spouses lives as well as being able to share with them what's happening in yours.

Are we giving kids too many options for their meals?

TABLE TOPICS

One of our favorite dinnertime games to play is Table Topics. It's a great way to engage your kids. They are a godsend to parents who want to engage their kids at the end of the day but are too tired to think of fun and creative conversation topics. There are some great diverse categories: specialty cards with questions for kids, travel, religion, and many others. Since moms and dads are sometimes— ok, usually—too tired to think up fun, creative and new topics every night, these conversation cards are a great way to engage the older as well as the younger kids. Even the adult set has questions that are easily answerable by a kindergartner. This will keep them at the table and eating bites between taking turns.

Sometimes the pressure of getting a child to try something new every night, or do the fourteen day repeat to introduce a veggie, can get stressful. Incorporating games into mealtime can help relieve some of that stress on everyone and take away part of the battle. The cards can be found on line (www.tabletopics.com), as well as in drugstores, toy stores and specialty stores.

Show-and-Tell

Both at home and anywhere else you go, you have a golden opportunity to play show-and-tell with food, especially at superstores like Costco, Super Target or Sam's Club, where there is a large selection of foods—even of organic options. Kids are highly visual. Ask them age appropriate questions about what they think are good and bad choices in each section of the store and why. Have them show you what foods they would choose and why. Many times, there are people also serving food samples, so this can make it even more fun. Turn it into a scored game: the one who makes the best choices, wins.

The Color Quiz

Walk children through the variety of colors found in fruits and veggies and talk about the specific nutrients that each color provides and which part of their bodies it's helping. You can make notecards or flashcards that your children can color to remember what each fruit and veggie does. Are the carrots helping their eyes? Are the red apples helping them sit still and concentrate? Is the calcium in the kale making their bones strong for soccer? Is the cantaloupe making their lungs stronger? Explain to them that by eating these fruits and veggies, not only will they feel better and do better in school, they will be able to stay away from the doctor's office—and that means fewer shots! It also means less medical spending for mom and dad in an economy where we are all watching our pennies.

Traffic Light Eating

This methodology for teaching kids how to make healthy choices was developed by Dr. William Sears. Assign foods a red light, yellow light or green light, depending on how often and how much of that food your child should be eating. That way, children can make educated choices in a fun way. They will understand the simplicity of red-yellow-green and can apply it easily when foods are clearly marked. Red light foods should be eaten in limited quantities. They are foods that are higher in sugar, fat or starch, like a hamburger or white pasta or heavy casserole dishes like King Ranch Chicken. Yellow light foods are lighter proteins, like tuna salad, three bean salad or roasted potatoes. The green light foods are things like hummus, guacamole and all fruits and vegetables. Play the traffic light game with your children at home, at restaurants or in the grocery store. Have them give each food a red, yellow or green light. The traffic light game is also a way to make them aware of the portions they should eat: how many fruits and vegetables versus meats and starches.

Lunch Time Prep

Print out the school cafeteria menu for the week. Talk to your kids about what's being served. Then you can play games and circle which foods they think they should pick out at school and which ones they like. This will also give you a better idea of what to serve at home that evening to balance out what they're eating for the day.

Use the internet: for kids who are old enough, set up parental controls and let them look up nutrients of different foods and play interactive games on sites like:

- http://www.nourishinteractive.com/kids/kidsarea.html

- http://www.nutritionexplorations.org/kids.php

- http://www.sheppardsoftware.com/nutritionforkids/games/foodgroupsgame.html

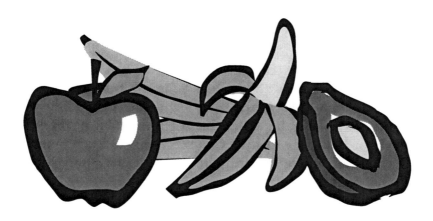

Involve and Include Your Children

Children are natural helpers. Encouraging your kids to cook and help out in the kitchen from an early age is great for creating healthy eating habits. Helping out in the kitchen also improves self-confidence and self-esteem and gives them a chance to develop what my family calls "life skills."

Most recently, our oldest daughter, who is in fifth grade, was asked by her science teacher to plan, prepare, cook and clean up after an entire meal on her own. She was amazing! She told me what to buy at the store and once she had the food proceeded to handle the entire meal without any help. She cooked, set the table, cleared and cleaned all on her own. All of our kids are capable of doing this on a regular basis, but how often do we ask them? Most of the time, we think it's just easier to do it ourselves. It's important that we turn to our kids to help them cultivate confidence and to reassure them that they can take care of themselves if necessary. And, we need a break as well!

Remember, being part of the cooking and preparation process is important for them and it also reduces your workload at the same time and fosters family togetherness. All it takes is one child helping to set the table and one child helping to make the salad to make a huge difference in your mealtime workload. For older children—tweens and teens—this tends to be a time where they open up and share thoughts about their day or things that might be bothering them. It's a perfect time to listen to them as they feel less inhibited and more prone to share since it's not a formal preplanned "talk."

Don't try to do it all for your kids. You will find that the more they help out in the morning and evening, the more time you will have to prepare a nutritious dinner for them. Stress the importance of working as a family team and reward their participation. Kids these days are becoming more and more entitled and are having a hard time coping in the real world as independent people once they leave home. You can give them many of the life skills they will need by offering them an opportunity to help out more at home—especially in the kitchen.

Cooking together creates closer bonds between parents and children and also between siblings. These are the memories they will look back on and smile.

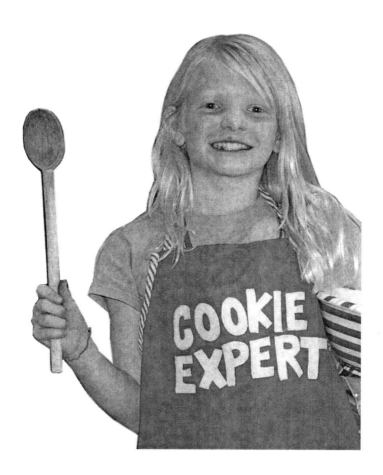

Research published in the *Journal of Epidemiology and Community Health* says children who have a diet high in fat, sugar and processed foods may have a lower IQ later in life. Remember, you child's brain is 90 percent formed around age five, so good nutrition is especially critical in the early years.

Kids Can Cook

Each child should learn to prepare one meal well, something that he or she can be proud of and make for the family as well as friends.

Remember to KISS (Keep It Simple Stupid, which was the name of a diet a co-worker of mine tried years ago). Let's be realistic here: your child does not need to become a French chef overnight, nor do you or your spouse. It's not about how fancy or complicated the meal is, or how many reduction sauces they can make. It's about health, exploration, autonomy and independence for your child—and eventually you.

Find out what they like, make sure it's healthy and provides a rainbow plate of nutrients, simplify it for them if necessary and then get them going. If you have several kids, this dramatically reduces your time in the kitchen. If you enjoy cooking and really want to participate yourself, even better. There's nothing more fun than developing a rhythm with someone in the kitchen and cooking together. It's a wonderful way to get some one-on-one quality time with a child or a spouse. Turn up the tunes and have a great time. But on their night, let them lead and pick their menu. Remember, it's their night, so you are not the executive chef; you are the sous-chef.

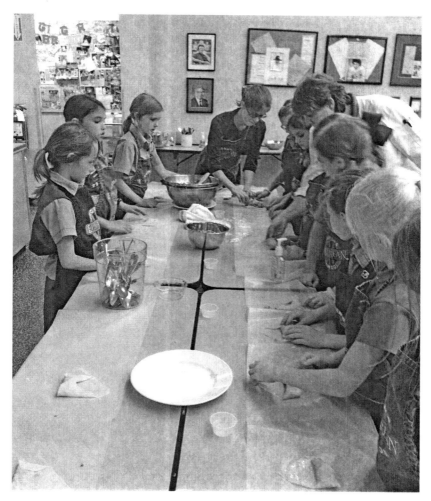

Have a tasting party and make the
preparation process fun!

EASY TWENTY-MINUTE MEALS

Easy meals like stir-fries are a wonderful way to serve slivers of different vegetables in a tangy sauce with your child's choice of meat, or you can go completely vegetarian. Kids love chicken, turkey, or pork-fried brown rice with cut up carrots, peas and onions and other fun Asian veggies like crunchy water chestnuts. Try making a stir-fry buffet where people can pick and choose which sauces, proteins and veggies they want in their stir-fry. If they're old enough let them chop stir-fries and sauces, design healthy, colorful pizzas. Most kids like dips. Slice up a variety of red, green, and yellow peppers along with carrots, celery, broccoli, cauliflower, cherry tomatoes, etc., and serve it with a dip or dressing that they like. For dessert, let the young ones arrange different colored berries and fruits on a tray.

Take the struggle out of trying new things and make it FUN. Kids are much more willing to try something new when they have been part of the preparation process or control it all together.

Team Clean

And don't forget the cleanup: mom—or dad—should NOT be prepping, cooking and cleaning up after every meal. This is not how things work in a family. It is perfectly normal for a nine-year-old to load the dishwasher after dinner and for a six-year-old to clear the table and help put away nonbreakables.

We have had kids over as guests who look at me like I am crazy when I ask them to take their plate to the kitchen. Parents, you are doing your kids a disservice if you don't teach them the simplest of life skills and you will totally wear yourselves out trying to do it all yourselves. Make them earn their keep. Kids will never develop a sense of self pride if everything is always done for them. Teach each child how to make a few simple meals and assign each of them one or two nights a week to do so—funny how quickly mom gets appreciated!

How Your Garden Grows

If you want to give your family a gift that will grow with them for life, then start a vegetable garden. There is no child that does not like to dig in the earth and everyone is moved by the miracle of tiny seeds growing into colorful, edible vegetables. If your children don't immediately appreciate the pleasure of eating these vegetables be patient. By gardening with your kids, you have started a personal connection between your children and the food they eat.

Turn the electronics off and go out as a family and begin the greatest bonding experience you can imagine. Share in the design, construction, sowing, the watering, watching and waiting, and finally the harvesting with your children. They will be much more likely to taste these homegrown vegetables whose readiness they have been anticipating and more likely to enjoy their fresher, tastier flavor. And, last but not least, encourage your children to take some over to their neighbors and friends. They will feel such a sense of pride when they see the surprise and admiration on their faces.

Help your kids grow a small garden—even a small herb garden works—to give them a better appreciation and understanding of where food actually comes from. Many children don't associate food in a fast-food bag or from a restaurant with something that actually comes out of the ground. I had a six-year-old child recently look at me like I was crazy when I told him that the baked chicken we were having for dinner was actually chicken! He had never seen it in any other form than a chicken nugget.

You don't even need a yard to garden, simply buy a few pots and throw in some soil and seasonal seeds and see what happens. My daughters' Pre-K class did this very haphazardly every year and had wonderful results! I was skeptical when I watched the kids throwing in seeds randomly, but it really does work.

We are now in a high-rise and my eleven-year-old daughter is trying to grow several different things inside. She has planted flaxseed, apple, tomato, cilantro and blackberries in plastic cups just to see what happens.

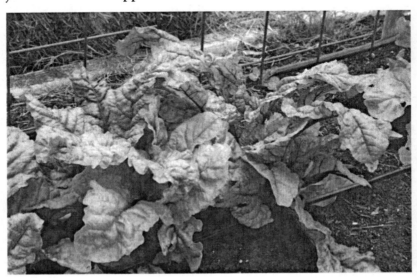

Why have we stopped eating seasonally when those seasonal fruits and vegetables are specifically designed by our creator to help our bodies meet the challenges of each particular season? Did you know that simply by adding some local and seasonal foods to your diet, your family will be better able to tolerate the changes and illnesses of each season?

If you live in an inner city and can't actually grow the food yourself, explore other options like joining a co-op, where you can get great local and season food.

FACT:
Nearly 1/3 of
kids in the
United States
eat fast food
every day.

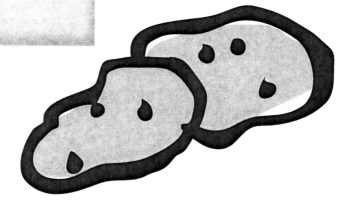

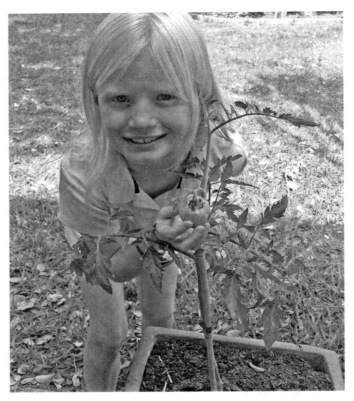

The Family Garden

Vegetables and fruits grow best in loose soil. One of the easiest ways to create a raised bed with good soil is to make a rectangular edge out of 2 x 12 boards. You can have them cut at your lumberyard to whatever size you want. It is all right, in fact better, to start out small. Place the boards together to form the rectangles and nail the boards together at the joining ends. Choose a sunny spot in your yard to place the rectangle. With a hoe or shovel remove all of the grass or weeds. Put the rectangle in the cleared spot and lay some crushed rocks in the bottom to help with draining. Buy enough organic soil to fill the rectangular area within two inches of the top.

Then comes the fun part. Go to your nearest plant and seed store and determine what can be planted at this time of year. You can buy seeds or sets that are ready to plant. Follow the directions about planting and watering. Then water as needed and watch it all happen.

If you do not have a yard area, pots and window boxes may be used. If none of these are available to you, then search out community gardens in your neighborhood and/or offer to start a garden at your children's school.

The wonderful thing about running your own vegetable garden is that you don't have to pick the produce until it is perfectly ripe. Most grocery stores sell produce that is picked before it is ready with the expectation that it will ripen in transit. But most fruits and vegetables that are prematurely picked never develop even close to their optimum flavor nor do they offer the same nutritional benefits. So, what do you have to lose? Start a little garden today. Your children will be captivated by the growing process. And they will be more eager to taste the food they have grown and will be more likely to truly enjoy the produce on their plate because it will taste better.

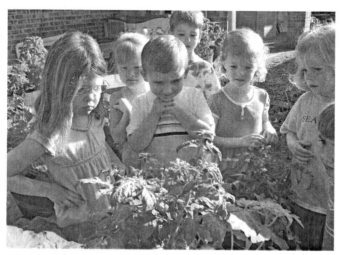

A small garden can produce big results

Shopping

To shop or not to shop, with or without kids—that is the question. Unfortunately, we are not all lucky enough to leave the kids behind when we go to the grocery store. But the truth is, taking one child with you can be a fun experience. When you start adding kids, it can get a bit more hairy, especially when they are young.

But remember, grocery shopping with your kids is a teachable moment at any age. As soon as they are able to eat "real" food, grocery shopping can become a fantastic way for you to share your views on food with your child and mold theirs for life.

How, you ask? Well, for the little ones, when you enter the store and they start reaching for food, do you offer them a piece of fruit or a bag of chips? What do they see you buying? Once again, you are modeling for your kids and have a chance to frame their views on food by what you purchase.

Shopping becomes a great teachable moment when you are able to converse with them about what's available in the store. You can teach them that the food they see on the perimeter of the store is different from what they see in the center aisles. You can ask them how it's different and why they think all the healthy food is on the edges of the store and everything in bags and boxes is on the center aisles. Teach them how to shop wisely. They'll remember.

You can talk about food marketing and look at why certain items are packaged the way they are. Why do the sugary cereals and salty chips target kids with cute box labels or bag designs? You can reinforce the importance of buying fresh produce and your kids will begin to see how many great options there are in the fruit and vegetable section. Introduce them to foods they wouldn't normally see, like a Daikon radish, and show them how fresh food is beautiful. You can also point out that the artificial colors they see in sports drinks and certain packaged snacks aren't part of the "real" food chain.

Shopping is also a great opportunity for experimenting with math and teaching budgets. Many stores have the opportunity for kids to weigh produce themselves, a wonderful chance to learn about units of measurement. You can also involve your children in the budget for each grocery trip. Have them add up what you are spending as you go to make sure you are on track. Make a game of it—at the register see how close their estimations are to the final bill.

Talk with your children about seasonality and why certain foods are less expensive and more available at certain times of the year. Explain to them that eating seasonally can keep you healthy, that specific foods grow at specific times of the year because they contain the nutrients your body needs for that season. Remind them that the nutrients found in whole, "real" foods are not going to be in an energy bar.

But beware: Don't let grocery shopping with kids undermine any progress you've made around eating. Do not give in to junk food requests. In the kitchen you are the boss and at the grocery store you are the boss. When the whining and pestering set in, it is another chance to put your parenting and behavioral skills to work. For example, when your kids are begging for a certain sugary snack or drink, your answer is, simply, "We don't eat that in our house."

The grocery store is a great platform for teaching nutrition and health to your kids. Use it to your advantage. There are different teaching benefits whether you are shopping in a large wholesale store or a small boutique grocery. The important thing to remember is that shopping, learning and eating is fun.

The Beginning

Rather than call this the end of the guide, I'd like to call it the beginning. I hope that the information I've shared with you has inspired you to make a new start with your family.

Everything I've shared—from statistics to personal and professional experiences—I've offered to give you hope.

In the first section, I explained the state of our nation when it comes to our children's health—where we've been but hopefully not where we're staying. To move forward, I believe you have to have a true understanding of what you're up against today. If we truly care about our children, it's time for radical change. I recently saw a quote up on the wall in my yoga class that said this:

"When the pain of being the same becomes greater than the pain of being different, you change"

> — Deepak Chopra, *Why Is God Laughing?: The Path to Joy and Spiritual Optimism*

This really hit home with me. But let's not wait until the pain is too great; let's do it now, before we get to a place of pain. If you are already there, then make the change.

In section two, I outlined what *not* to feed your family and hopefully shed some light on supplementation and ways to make up for what's missing in our food supply. Take the time to read labels and bring up the level of food awareness in your family. Seek out real food and help your kids learn to make choices that will keep them (and their own children one day) healthy for life. Food has changed; we have to change as well.

In the final section, I gave you the tools you need to implement change in your home. Behavior modification—breaking old habits and starting fresh—will be the key to your success. I invite you to make a commitment to a *new viewpoint* and a *new way* of doing things both in your home and on the go. Will it be any easier than the way you've done things in the past? Not necessarily. But the results are more than worth the effort.

When you attempt anything new, it seems difficult. But if you give it some thought you'll realize it's only tough because you have grown accustomed to doing things the old way and it feels uncomfortable to change. The reality is, it's not harder, it's simply different.

Not only do you need to change your actions but you need to change your perspective.

"If you only change what you do, all you get are temporary changes to your actions. Change your inner viewpoint, though, and your world transforms."[17]

It's time to change our view of food, health and eating. As parents, we have the opportunity to positively impact our children's lives every single day. They are sponges, watching us, listening to us, ready and waiting for whatever we have to offer.

What message are you sending? What lessons are you teaching daily? What patterns and habits are you willing to break to reclaim your child's health? Is your child going to be the one to break free from years of family obesity or continue down the road of ill health your family has been on for several generations?

Ultimately, the choice is yours. As a parent, you are a healer. I've given you the information you need to start today. The rest is up to you.

Rainbow Recipes

Spicy Healthy Lemonade . . . an alternative to juice!

- 8 oz. cool purified water
- 1-2 tbsp. honey
- 1-2 tbsp. Bragg's Apple Cider Vinegar (to taste)

Tricolor Pepper Omelet with Ezekiel Toast

- Organic red, green, yellow or orange bell peppers*
- 1/4 diced onion
- Organic or cage-free eggs
- 1 tsp. ghee or olive oil
- Nitrate-free bacon or turkey sausage (optional)
- Ezekiel toast or Ezekiel English muffin
- Sea salt or rock salt and pepper to taste

In a separate pan, lightly sauté onions and peppers in ghee (see sidebar) or olive oil. Scramble eggs with sea salt and pepper to taste. Pour into an omelet pan and add veggies and crumbled bacon or turkey sausage. Serve with a side of Ezekiel toast with a dab of homemade ghee!

*Remember to try and buy organic peppers when you can since they are one of the Dirty Dozen!

Power-Packed Smoothie

- Strawberries

- Kale

- Blueberries

- Honey

- Organic ground flax (or hemp seeds or krill oil*)

- Banana

- Unsweetened Yogurt (optional)

*You can also substitute 1 tsp. of a plant-based oil like BodyBio-Balance (www. bodybio.com) made from organic sunflower and flax oils. It has the perfect 4:1 ratio of omega 6:3 and the kids might prefer this as there is no fish taste since it's plant based.

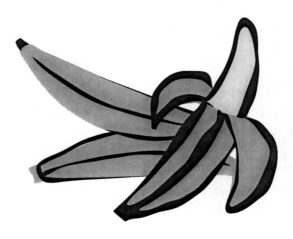

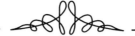

Four-Grain Pancakes Served with Homemade Applesauce

- 1/4 cup organic whole wheat flour
- 1/4 cup organic white flour
- 1/6 cup organic cornmeal (try blue cornmeal too)
- 1 rounded tbsp. rolled oatmeal
- 1 tsp. organic brown sugar
- 1/4 tsp. salt
- Dash of cinnamon
- 1/3 tsp. baking soda
- 1 tsp. baking powder
- 1 1/2 tbsp. melted butter
- 2 tbsp. honey
- Slightly over 1/2 cup milk

Mix all together. Heat pancake skillet over medium heat. Rub 1 tsp. unsalted butter or a little canola oil on a paper towel over the pancake skillet. Drop a large tbsp. of mixture on to heated skillet. Spread out a little. Cook until underside is brown. Flip pancakes and cook until they are done. From 1 to 1-1/2 minutes per pancake. Serve with organic maple syrup slightly warmed and homemade applesauce.

Serves 4.

Adapted from the *Joy of Cooking*

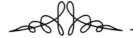

Blueberry Yogurt Pancakes for Two

- 1/2 cup organic unbleached flour
- 1/8 tsp. baking soda
- 1/4 tsp. baking powder
- Pinch of salt
- 1 free-range organic egg
- 3 tbsp. water
- 2 tbsp. melted organic butter
- 1/2 cup organic blueberries
- 1 3.7-ounce bottle of Siggi's probiotic drinkable nonfat blueberry yogurt

Mix the dry ingredients together. Add the egg, yogurt, butter and water. Stir in the blueberries (These may be left out if you want the pancakes plain or add your favorite chopped nuts or alternative fruit.) Heat a pancake skillet under medium-high heat for 2 minutes. Very lightly butter the surface of the pan (1 tsp. of butter).

When pan is hot ladle pancake mixture onto the pan for five pancakes. Cook until medium dark on first side. Flip and cook new side to same amount. When cooking with whole, refrigerated blueberries, you have to be sure the pancake is cooked throughout. Serve with 100% Vermont maple syrup or honey. You can double or triple this recipe as needed.

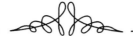

Easy One-Dish Baked Chicken

- 4 chicken legs and 4 chicken thighs
- Olive oil
- 1 large lemon
- 1 small purple onion cut in 1-inch pieces
- 2 garlic cloves finely chopped
- 1 ripe organic tomato cut into eighths and then each slice halved
- 4 organic new potatoes cut in quarters
- 1/2 cup olives pitted (optional)
- 1/2 tsp. dried poultry seasoning
- 1/4 cup fresh basil
- One 4-sprig of fresh rosemary cut in four pieces
- 1 package young fresh asparagus: take the lower six inches and cut into three sections. If the asparagus are thick then you will have to peel them or they will be too tough. You could also use sliced zucchini.
- 4 slices of prosciutto cut in thirds.
- Salt and pepper to taste.
- Juice of one lemon.

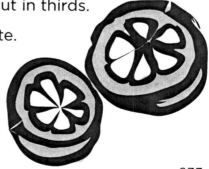

Use a sided baking sheet or a large rectangular Pyrex baking dish. Pour 1/4 cup olive oil into the baking dish. Place the chicken pieces, onions and potatoes in the dish, stir them around to fully coat in the olive oil. Salt and pepper to taste. Sprinkle with 1/2 tsp. dried poultry seasoning. Place tomatoes, olives and garlic on top of the chicken. Then top with the prosciutto and drizzle a little olive oil over them. Sprinkle some salt and pepper over the entire mixture. This dish may be prepared up to three hours ahead of time and kept covered in the refrigerator. Bring to room temperature before baking.

Bake in a 375 degree oven for 30 minutes. Turn the chicken and other ingredients over at least once. Add the asparagus and bake for another 2-3 minutes or until the chicken is done. If you want the chicken browned a little then broil the dish for the last 10 minutes, watching carefully not to burn any of it.

Serves 6-8.

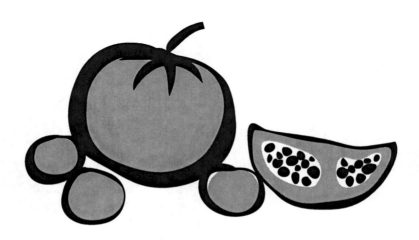

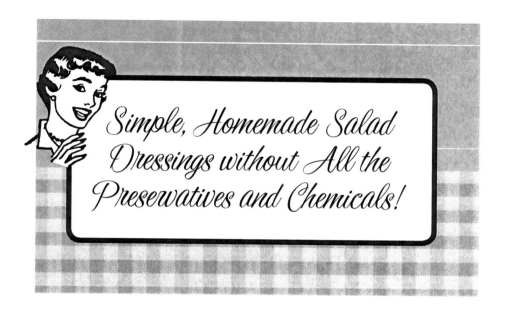

Simple, Homemade Salad Dressings without All the Preservatives and Chemicals!

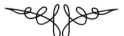

Ethel's Easy Vinaigrette

- 1/2 cup olive oil
- 1/3 cup Bragg's Apple Cider Vinegar
- 1/2 to 1 tsp. finely chopped garlic
- Salt and pepper to taste

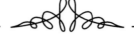

Cilantro Vinaigrette

Place in a blender:

- 1/2 cup olive oil

- 1/3 cup apple cider vinegar

- 1 clove chopped garlic

- 1 tbsp. organic honey

- 1 handful chopped cilantro

- Salt and pepper to taste

Puree briefly.

This is a great dressing to serve over frisée lettuce, mixed greens or butter lettuces along with thinly julienned mangoes, julienned cooked beets, crumbled goat cheese and pistachios. YUM! (Adapted from the house salad at Indika, Houston, Texas)

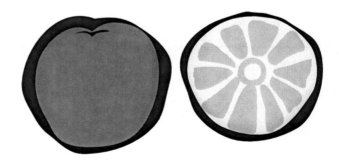

Melissa's Nantucket Blueberry Dressing

Place in blender:

- 1/2 cup olive oil

- 1/3 cup balsamic vinegar

- 1/2 cup blueberries

- Salt and pepper to taste

Most tasty served with spinach salad, fresh organic blueberries, pecans and crumbled blue cheese. This recipe was taken from Post Oak Grill, a restaurant of Ethel's in Houston. Her pastry chef Melissa Piper came up with it and it was one of her best sellers!

Light and Crisp Citrus dressing

- 1/2 cup olive oil

- 1/4 cup fresh squeezed orange juice

- 1 tbsp. fresh lemon juice

- Salt and pepper to taste

This dressing is best served with a mixture of watercress and lettuce, thinly sliced radishes and fennel, and fresh orange sections. You can also add fresh, wild grilled salmon for extra protein or shrimp and jumbo lump crab.

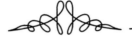

Mango Mustard Dressing

Place in blender

- 1/2 cup olive oil

- 1/2 cup white balsamic vinegar

- 1/2 cup chopped mango

- 2 tsp. Dijon mustard

- 1 garlic clove chopped

- 1/4 cup chopped Italian parsley

- Salt and freshly ground pepper to taste

Puree briefly.

Mango mustard dressing tastes wonderful with a salad of red tipped lettuce, avocado, sliced apple and walnuts. You can add natural grilled chicken for extra protein or to make it a heavier meal.

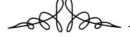

Turkey Scallops

Thirty years ago my cousin in London was able to buy thin slices of turkey which she cooked for her children like you would cook veal. It was inexpensive, delicious and easy to cook. Whole Foods is now selling them.

- 4 turkey scallops

- 2 tbsp. clarified butter (ghee) olive oil or butter. Clarified butter or ghee is easy to make. Just heat the butter until it separates. The solids will stay in the bottom of the pan. Use the clear butter liquid to cook with. The solids are the part that will clog your arteries, but the clear liquid remaining still imparts a delicious buttery flavor.

- Juice of 1 lemon

Put the clarified butter in the skillet. Cook the scallops on both sides on medium high heat until cooked through. Remove from the skillet and turn the skillet on low. Add the juice of one lemon. Stir with the remaining butter. Return the turkey scallops to the skillet and swirl them around in the lemon butter.

Serve with either a baked new or sweet potato and sugar snap peas. This is a colorful, nutritious and delicious dinner that takes no time.

Bake four red new potatoes or four small sweet potatoes baked in the oven until tender. This takes about 30 minutes in a 450 degree oven, depending on the size of the potatoes.

Lightly steam two cups of sugar snap peas. They should still be crunchy.

Serves 4

Note: this same dish can be made with wild tilapia or flounder filets.

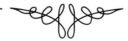

Gabrielle White Bean Chicken Stew

- 1 box organic (32 oz.) chicken or veggie broth

- 2 small cans of diced green chilis (you can do mild or spicy, to taste)

- 2 pulled all-natural or organic chicken breasts. You can also substitute ham or nitrate-free sausage

- 2 cans white navy beans, Great Northern beans or Cannellini, or any other white bean, rinsed

- 1/2 onion

- 4 cloves garlic

- 1 tbsp. Herbs de Provence to taste (this is a spice combination of French herbs found at all grocery stores, but it is optional)

- Salt to taste

Sprinkle chicken with salt and pepper and sauté chicken breasts. Let cool. Open beans, rinse and let drain in colander. Lightly cook onions in 2 tbsps. ghee or olive oil, then add garlic for 30 seconds. Add one pinch of salt and the Herbs de Provence. Add beans and chilis to onion and garlic mixture and then add chicken broth. Turn to boil and while waiting, pull chicken into shreds, then add to the pot. Boil for 1 minute then simmer for flavors to come together.

Will feed 4 and is great served with homemade jalapeno cheese corn bread! Serving time: 20 minutes.

Black Bean Summer Salad

- 1 can rinsed organic corn
- 1 can rinsed organic black beans
- 1 peeled cucumber cut into small squares
- 1 container feta cheese
- 2 chopped tomatoes
- 1/2 chopped purple onion
- Chopped cilantro to taste
- Mix with Ethel's Easy Vinaigrette

This will serve 4-6 people as a side for grilling out or at a barbeque, or simply by itself!

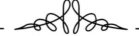

Easiest Ever Pasta with Tomato Sauce

- 2 14-oz. cans of crushed fire roasted tomatoes
- 3-4 cloves of fresh garlic peeled and finely chopped
- Organic olive oil
- 1/2 cup pitted black olives
- 1 tsp. dried oregano
- 1/4-1/2 tsp. Italian dried red pepper flakes
- Salt and pepper to taste
- Whole grain spaghetti

Sauté lightly the garlic in three tablespoons of olive oil. Add the canned tomatoes and simmer with lid on for 5 minutes. Add the black olives. Add the oregano, salt and pepper, and red pepper flakes and simmer on low with the lid on for 5-10 minutes. Cook the whole grain pasta according to directions until al dente. Add some cooking water for the pasta to the sauce if it is too thick. Drain the pasta. Serve immediately with the tomato sauce.

Feeds 4-6 kids.

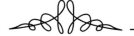

Sautéed Julienne Vegetables, Camille's Way!

- 2 zucchini

- 2 yellow squash

- 2 carrots

- 2 tbsps. organic butter, clarified butter (ghee) or olive oil

- 1/4 tsp. ground thyme

- Salt and pepper to taste

Julienne or cut in slivers the yellow squash, zucchini and squash. Stir-fry the vegetables very slightly in butter or olive oil over high heat. Be careful not to overcook them. They should be a little brown but not soft. Add salt, pepper and thyme. Serve immediately or they will become soggy.

Serves 4-6.

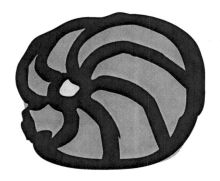

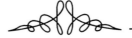

Sautéed Sugar Snap Peas with Prosciutto and Onion

- 2 cups sugar snap peas (fresh spring peas are good also)

- 1/4 cup chopped yellow onions

- 1/4 cup chopped prosciutto. The prosciutto should not be too thin or it is difficult to chop

- 2 tbsp. olive oil

Sauté the onions and prosciutto in a pan over medium heat until the onions are soft. Add the peas and sauté until slightly cooked but still crisp. Salt and pepper to taste. Serve immediately. For a slightly different version add thin strips of red or yellow bell pepper with the peas.

Serves 4-6.

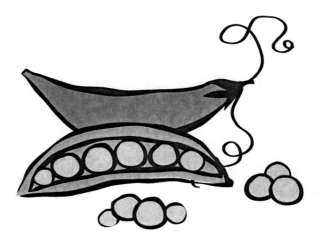

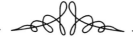

Elida's Easy Green Chile Chicken Enchiladas*

- 1 baked chicken, no skin**
- 1 5.3-oz. container Greek Yogurt (I like Oikos by Stoneyfield Farms) or nonfat sour cream
- 2 16-oz. packages shredded Monterey Jack or Mexican blend cheese
- 1 33-oz. jar Green Chile Stew Mix
- 30 corn tortillas
- 1 cup chicken broth

Preheat oven to 325 degrees. Pull chicken meat from chicken into shreds and drop into mixing bowl with the ¾ stew mix, one packet of the cheese and all of the Greek Yogurt.

Heat the chicken broth in a small sauté pan.

Individually dip corn tortillas into warm broth, then remove. Fill with as much or as little of the chicken filling as you choose. If you use 2 tbsp., your mixture will go further but you will have smaller enchiladas. Fill the tortilla, wrap it and set it lengthwise in a rectangular glass dish. Repeat until the dishes are full. You should be able to fill two dishes.

Top off dish with remaining cheese and reserved green chili stew mix. You can add Greek yogurt as well.

Cook until cheese is melted and bubbling.

Top it off with some salsa and homemade guacamole for a yummy feast.

*This is a great meal for parties! The trays will feed 15-20 people and these also freeze really well.

**The recipe can also be made substituting shrimp for the chicken and you can add canned black beans and or corn to give the enchiladas a bit more substance.

Fifteen-Minute Stir-Fry

There are two ways to go about making this dish. You can buy frozen stir-fry veggies which work well when you're running in late from sports and don't have time to prep food. I like to keep these in my fridge all the time for back up. Or you can slice and dice your own mixture.

In addition, you can vary the meat or use none at all. You can use pork, beef, chicken or shrimp: they all make for a great stir-fry!

I am going to give you several options and a list of many ingredients you can cut up and add. The beauty of stir-fry is that it's quick and you really can use whatever you have in your fridge or pantry: there is not a set ingredient list!

- 3 tbsp. sesame, canola or peanut oil
- 2 chopped garlic cloves
- 1 cup snow peas
- 1 cup bok choy (optional)
- 1/2 cup chopped celery
- 1/2 white onion or 1/2 cup green onions
- 1 cup mixed, sliced bell peppers
- 1 can water chestnuts, drained
- 1/4 cup cashews
- 2 garlic cloves
- Soy sauce
- Red chili pepper flakes (optional for spice)

- Fresh grated and chopped ginger (optional: you can also use powdered)

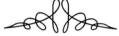

For stir-fry sauce:

- 1/4 cup brown sugar

- 1 tbsp. minced fresh ginger root

- 2 lg. cloves garlic, minced

- 1/2 tsp. ground red pepper

- 1/2 cup soy sauce

- 1/4 cup cider or rice wine vinegar

Cube and cook whatever your meat choice was in the oil and set aside. If it's shrimp, peel before cooking. You can leave tails on or remove them. Add more oil to the pan and throw in remaining veggies on high heat. Stir for 5 minutes. You want veggies to remain crisp. Reserve the garlic until the last 30 seconds as it cooks quickly, then add to pan. Add your chicken, shrimp, pork or beef at this time as well.

To make a great sauce, mix all the above stir-fry sauce ingredients together and add to final mixture. Stir for one minute then you're done!

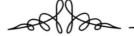

Ethel's Easy Chicken Salad

- 4 cups cubed (1/2 inch) cooked chicken (about 1 3/4 pound)
- 1 cup walnuts or pecans, chopped
- 2 tbsps. finely chopped shallot
- 2 cups halved seedless red grapes
- 3/4 cup Greek yogurt
- 3 tbsps. tarragon or red wine vinegar
- 1/2 tsp. salt
- 1/2 tsp. black pepper

Mix all ingredients together and serve on a bed of baby mixed greens with rice crackers, flax or whole grain crackers. Or better yet, you can use Nut Thins, one of my favorite crackers. This is a great meal to take to the office or on a picnic.

Feeds 4-6.

Acknowledgments

They say it takes a village to raise a child. Well, it also takes a village to publish a book!

This has been an incredible process, both exhilarating and exhausting from the very start, and I am incredibly grateful to everyone who has been so patient with me. For you moms out there, you know that there are only so many hours a day to get things done and the physical and emotional needs of your family are always there. Thanks to everyone that got me through and thanks to my husband and kids for their patience!

My brother, Kirksey, started the ball rolling on this whole book-writing process after my first appearance on *Great Day Houston* by saying to me "Now you're going to have to write a book!" I laughed at him, hung up the phone, and twenty-four hours later I started writing. Why? Because the idea scared the heck out of me, which told me that it was the right thing to do. I knew that I had to get my message out to all the parents who need help.

Most of all, I want to thank my husband, Rallin, and my three girls. You've been my guinea pigs and my strongest supporters.

I am so grateful for my parents, Ethel and Ray, who raised me to love good, clean food with the organic garden we had growing up, and my stepparents Chap and Zulay for their continued support. Mom, thank you for being my coauthor and partner in this from the beginning and encouraging me to push forward. You have so much knowledge!

Thanks so much to my team of superstars and supporters who encouraged me and then got me off the ground: Stacey Morgenstern, Beth Lambert, Beth Aldrich, Robin O'Brien and Sonya Wilson.

I adore my incredibly patient and creative design team at MacGraphics Design: Kerrie Lian, Karen Saunders and Helena Mariposa. You guys are amazing.

Thank you to Mary Walewski with buythebookmarketing. com who has helped me get *The Pizza Trap* out there and taught me that social media is my friend.

Patrice Rhoades-Baum, the queen of branding, you are the best!

Dr. Devinder Bhatia, thank you for your medical foreword and your support of my endeavor from day one as a mutual health warrior and friend.

Last, but definitely not least, thanks to my editor, Marisa Belger, who has been working with me on this for a couple of years now. None of this would have been possible without your insight, editing skills and persistence; not to mention pulling ideas out of me I didn't even realize were there.

We did it!

Notes

Introduction

1. A. Branum and S. Lukacs, "Food Allergy Among US Children: Trends in Prevalence and Hospitalization," *National Center for Health Statistics Data Brief*, 10, October 2008.

2. Pediatrics study: http://pediatrics.aappublications.org/content/early/2012/05/15/peds.2011-1082.abstract.

3. http://www.clinicalepigeneticsjournal.com/content/4/1/6/abstract.

4. http://ajrccm.atsjournals.org/content/183/4/441.short.

5. http://www.health.harvard.edu/newsletters/Harvard_Mental_Health_Letter/2009/June/Diet-and-attention-deficit-hyperactivity-disorder.

Section 1

1. Yale University Rudd Center for Food Policy and Obesity, "Cereal FACTS," http://www.yaleruddcenter.org/rudd-center-launches-update-on-cereal-facts.

2. Eric M. Bost, Undersecretary, "Food, Nutrition and Consumer Services," (US Dept of Agriculture, September 15, 2004).

3. *JAMA* 2003; 290:1884-1890.

4. Robert H. Lustig, MD, UCSF Professor of Pediatrics in the Division of Endocrinology, *Sugar—The Bitter Truth*, Health and Medicine, Show ID: 16717, (UCSF Mini Medical School for the Public, 7/2009).

5. American Heart Association, Monday April 9, 2012, http://www.heart.org/HEARTORG/GettingHealthy/Overweight-in-Children_UCM_304054_Article.jsp.

6. www.allergykids.com.

7. Ibid.

8. http://www.med.umich.edu/yourchild/topics/tv.htm, University of Michigan Health System; http://www.limitv.org/health.htm.

9. HBO: "The Weight of the Nation," part 1, http://www.youtube.com/watch?v=-pEkCbqN4uo.

10. http://aces.nmsu.edu/pubs/research/dairy/TR-42.pdf.

11. Patrick Holford, *The New Optimum Nutrition Bible* (New York: Crossing Press, 2005), 63.

12. William Mayo, founder Mayo Clinic.

13. Patrick Holford, *The New Optimum Nutrition Bible* (New York: Crossing Press, 2005), 56.

14. http://www.peta.org/

15. Steve Boyan, PhD, "How Our Food Choices can Help Save the Environment," http://www.earthsave.org/environment/foodchoices.htm.

16. http://www.wired.com/wiredscience/2008/11/fast-food-anoth/.

17. US Public Interest Research Group, http://www.uspirg.org/issues/usp/stop-subsidizing-obesity.

18. Physicians Committee for Responsible Medicine, http://www.pcrm.org/media/commentary/. For further information see: http://theweek.com/article/index/218167/americarsquos-food-deserts.

19. Ibid.

20. US Department of Agriculture (USDA).

21. Mary Sanchez, "Project Addresses Pesticide Risks among Migrant Workers," *The Kansas City Star*, January 23, 2003, B8.

22. California Department of Food and Agriculture.

23. Mount Sinai Medical Center, NYC, 1997.

Section 2

1. http://www.msgtruth.org.

2. Dr. Russell Blaylock, "Excitotoxins—The Taste That Kills," http://insuranceandwellness.com/Excitotoxins. pdf.

3. http://www.health.harvard.edu/blog/ astounding-increase-in-antidepressant-use-by-americans-201110203624.

4. Dr. William Sears and Dr. Peter Sears, *Dr. Sears' LEAN Kids*, (New York: New American Library, 2003), 26-44.

5. American Cancer Society, 1986; Qing Yang, "Gain Weight by 'Going Diet?' Artificial Sweeteners and the Neurobiology of Sugar Cravings," *Yale Journal of Biology and Medicine*, June 2010, 83 (2), 101-108, http://www. ncbi.nlm.nih.gov/pmc/articles/PMC2892765/.

6. www.livestrong.com/article/314167-the-effects-of-diet-cola/; Patrick Holford, *The New Optimum Nutrition Bible*, (Pennsylvania: Crossing Press, 2005).

7. Beth Greer, *Super Natural Home,* (New York: Rodale Books, 2009).

8. http://articles.mercola.com/sites/articles/
    archive/2009/04/21/msg-is-this-silent-killer-lurking-
    in-your-kitchen-cabinets.aspx; Russell L. Blaylock, MD,
    Excitotoxins: The Taste That Kills, (New Mexico: The
    Health Press, 1996).

9. http://envirocancer.cornell.edu/bibliography/general/
    bib.parabens.cfm; http://www.mayoclinic.com/health/
    stress/SR00001; http://www.healthguidance.org/
    entry/15893/1/List-of-Human-Hormones-and-Their-
    Importance.html.

10. http://www.organicauthority.com/blog/organic/breast-
    cancer-study-finds-parabens-in-virtually-all-tumors/#s.
    abti3vlyabaaa.

11. http://www.cdc.gov/chronicdisease/pdf/2009-power-of-
    prevention.pdf.

12. http://www.hsph.harvard.edu/nutritionsource/what-
    should-you-eat/fats-full-story/; http://www.ncbi.nlm.
    nih.gov/pubmed/11759276.

13. http://www.responsibletechnology.org/gmo-dangers/
    health-risks/articles-about-risks-by-jeffrey-smith/
    Genetically-Engineered-Foods-May-Cause-Rising-
    Food-Allergies-Genetically-Engineered-Soybeans-May-
    2007#endnote_1; Charles Sheehan, "Scientists See Spike
    in Kids' Food Allergies," *Chicago Tribune*, 9 June 2006;
    http://www.montereyherald.com/mld/montereyherald/
    living/health.

14. Mark Hyman, MD, *The UltraMind Solution: Fix Your
    Broken Brain by Healing Your Body First*, (New York:
    Scribner, 2010).

15. Robert H. Lustig, MD, UCSF Professor of Pediatrics in the Division of Endocrinology, *Sugar—The Bitter Truth*, Health and Medicine, Show ID: 16717, (UCSF Mini Medical School for the Public, 7/2009).

16. Ibid.

17. Ibid.

18. Dr. William Sears and Dr. Peter Sears, *Dr. Sears' LEAN Kids*, (New York: New American Library, 2003), 43-44.

19. Ibid., 31.

20. www.responsibletechnology.org.

21. Ibid.

22. Robert H. Lustig, MD, UCSF Professor of Pediatrics in the Division of Endocrinology, *Sugar—The Bitter Truth*, Health and Medicine, Show ID: 16717, (UCSF Mini Medical School for the Public, 7/2009).

23. http://www.cancer.org/Cancer/ CancerCauses/OtherCarcinogens/ GeneralInformationaboutCarcinogens/known-and-probable-human-carcinogens.

24. *Food Chemicals Codex* (3rd addition), (Washington: National Academy Press, 1992); http://nutritionfacts. org/video/meat-additives-to-diminish-toxicity/.

25. Dr. Kenneth Bock, *Healing the New Childhood Epidemics*, (New York: Ballantine Books, 2008).

26. pedersonfarms.com.

27. http://www.ncbi.nlm.nih.gov/pubmed/16550597.

28. http://www.livestrong.com/article/485372-side-effects-of-sodium-sulfite/#ixzz1tXvqVlZB.

29. Center for Science in the Public Interest, Jun 29, 2010.

30. University of Southampton. "Food Additives Linked to Hyperactivity in Children, Study Shows," *ScienceDaily*, September 10, 2007, http://www.sciencedaily.com/releases/2007/09/070909202847.htm.

31. http://www.organicauthority.com/foodie-buzz/what-is-in-fast-food-chicken-hint-its-not-chicken.html.

32. Dr. William Sears and Dr. Peter Sears, *Dr. Sears' LEAN Kids*, (New York: New American Library, 2003), 52.

33. www.thehealthyboy.com.

34. www.chemicalfreelife.tumblr.com.

35. http://www.all4naturalhealth.com/benefits-of-organic-food.html.

36. www.nordicnaturals.com; http://www.hsph.harvard.edu/nutritionsource/questions/omega-3/index.html.

37. Dr. Mark Hyman, *The UltraMind Solution: Fix Your Broken Brain by Healing Your Body First,* (New York: Scribner, 2010); http://probiotics.mercola.com/probiotics.html.

38. http://www.ncbi.nlm.nih.gov/pubmed/20029821.

39. http://michaelpollan.com/books/in-defense-of-food/.

40. https://www.princeton.edu/greening/organic4.htm.

41. http://www.fda.gov/downloads/ForIndustry/UserFees/AnimalDrugUserFeeActADUFA/UCM231851.pdf.

42. Jeannette Bessinger and Tracee Yablon-Blenner, *Simple Food for Busy Families,* (New York: Celestial Arts, 2009).

43. Jeannette Bessinger and Tracee Yablon-Blenner, *Simple Food for Busy Families,* (New York: Celestial Arts, 2009); Joshua Rosenthal, *Integrative Nutrition* (New York: Integrative Nutrition Publishing, 2008).

Section 3

1. http://www.upi.com/Health_News/2011/09/15/ Kids-who-play-sports-apt-to-be-overweight/UPI- 22011316059316/.

2. http://www.cdc.gov/obesity/data/childhood.html.

3. http://www.ncbi.nlm.nih.gov/pubmed/20059703.

4. http://www.childrensdefense.org/policy-priorities/ childrens-health/child-nutrition/childhood-obesity. html.

5. http://www.childrensdefense.org/policy-priorities/ childrens-health/child-nutrition/childhood-obesity. html.

6. http://www.ncbi.nlm.nih.gov/pmc/articles/ PMC1637197/; http://www.splendaexposed.com/.

7. http://www.cnn.com/2012/04/27/health/soda-obesity/ index.html?hpt=hp_c2.

8. http://www.cdc.gov/about/grand-rounds/ archives/2010/06-June.htm.

9. Dr. Sylvia Rimm, *Rescuing the Emotional Lives of Overweight Children*, (New York: Rodale, March 31, 2004).

10. Marion Nestle, *What to Eat*, (New York: North Point Press, 2006), 383.

11. http://www.time.com/time/magazine/article/0,9171,1200760,00.html#ixzz2780ofoa0.

12. http://www.time.com/time/magazine/article/0,9171,1200760,00.html#ixzz2780Djxqc.

13. http://www.ucsf.edu/news/2012/02/11437/societal-control-sugar-essential-ease-public-health-burden.

14. Alexander Wolff, "The New Training Table," *Sports Illustrated*, November 7, 2011.

15. http://www.huffingtonpost.com/dr-mark-hyman/how-to-get-rid-of-acne-pi_b_225057.html.

16. http://children.webmd.com/news/20101021/obesity-in-kids-rises-around-the-world.

17. Baron Baptiste, *Journey Into Power: How to Sculpt Your Ideal Body, Free Your True Self, and Transform Your Life With Yoga*, (New York: Simon & Schuster, 2002).

About the Authors

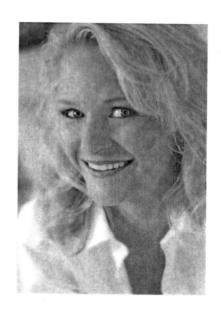

Gabrielle Welch

Gabrielle is a Certified Holistic Health Coach from the Institute for Integrative Nutrition. She holds a Nutritional Consultant degree from The Global College of Natural Medicine and is a Dr. Sears' L.E.A.N. certified Health Coach. She also has an MBA from Baylor University.

Gabrielle is a well-known public speaker who is featured regularly on Channel 11's *Great Day Houston* with Deborah Duncan and on The Live Well Network's *Deals* (ABC). She is also the founder of Welch Wellness, which educates, supports and inspires women and children to help prevent disease and embrace a life of wellness through nutrition, green living and life balance. Gabrielle's passion is to empower moms like herself with the knowledge to make better choices when it comes to cooking, buying groceries, choosing natural products for their home and families, and especially eating on-the-go.

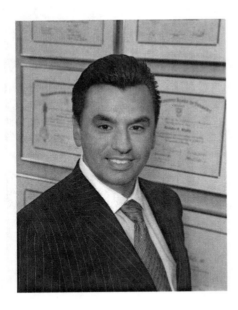

Dr. Devinder Bhatia

Dr. Devinder Bhatia, a renowned cardiovascular and thoracic surgeon, has authored or coauthored over twenty publications and is often sought out by television news programs to provide medical commentary. He was a guest speaker on the *Dr. Oz Show* and has been featured on several local news broadcasts.

Dr. Bhatia is board certified by the American Board of Thoracic Surgery and is a member of over twenty medical societies and organizations. He is particularly passionate about children's health and works to bring awareness to diet-related diseases affecting young people today—specifically obesity, diabetes and hypertension.

Dr. Bhatia currently practices in Houston and is a happily married father of three.

Bibliography

Baker, Nena. *The Body Toxic*. New York: North Point Press, 2008.

Bessinger, Jeannette, and Tracee Yablon-Brenner. *Simple Food for Busy Families*. Berkeley: Celestial Arts, 2009.

Bock, Dr. Kenneth, and Cameron Stauth. *Healing the New Childhood Epidemics*. New York: Ballantine Books, 2008.

Day, Phillip. *Health Wars*. Kent: Credence, 2001.

DesMaisons, Kathleen. *Little Sugar Addicts*. New York: Three Rivers Press, 2004.

Dorfman, Kelly. *What's Eating Your Child?* New York: Workman Publishing, 2011.

Ettlinger, Steve. *Twinkie Deconstructed*. New York: Penguin Group, 2007.

Fay, Jim. *Parenting with Love and Logic*. Golden: Love and Logic Press, 2006.

Glenn, H. Stephen, and Jane Nelsen. *Raising Self-Reliant Children in a Self-Indulgent World*. Roseville: Prima Publishing, 2000.

Greer, Beth. *Super Natural Home*. New York: Rodale, 2009.

Holford, Patrick. *The New Optimum Nutrition Bible*. New York: Crossing Press, 2004.

Hyman, Dr. Mark. *The UltraMind Solution: Fix Your Broken Brain by Healing Your Body First*. New York: Scribner, 2009.

Lambert, Beth. *A Compromised Generation*. Boulder: Sentient Publications, 2010.

Nestle, Marion. *What to Eat*. New York: North Point Press, 2007.

O'Brien, Robyn. *The Unhealthy Truth*. New York: Broadway, 2009.

Pollan, Michael. *In Defense of Food*. New York: Penguin, 2009.

Robin, Marie-Monique. *The World According to Monsanto*. New York: The New Press, 2010.

Rosenthal, Joshua. *Integrative Nutrition*. New York: Integrative Nutrition Publishing, 2008.

Schlosser, Eric. *Fast Food Nation*. New York: HarperCollins, 2001.

Sears, Dr. William. *The Healthiest Kid in the Neighborhood*. New York: Little, Brown and Company, 2006.

Sears, Dr. William. *The NDD Book*. New York: Little, Brown, and Company, 2009.

Smith, Jeffery. *Seeds of Deception*. Fairfield: Yes! Books, 2003.

Winter, Ruth. *A Consumer's Dictionary of Food Additives*. New York: Three Rivers Press, 2009.

Wu, Sarah. *Fed Up with Lunch*. San Francisco: Chronicle Books, 2011.

artificial sugars, 81, 136. *See also* artificial sweeteners; sugar substitutes

artificial sweeteners, 53, 55, 84, 136, 163

Asian veggies, 218. *See also* bok choy

asparagus, 99, 127, 141, 145, 154, 233–234

aspartame, 53–57, 58, 59, 75, 81, 95, 163

aspartic acid, 53

asthma, 1, 6, 7, 23, 24, 70, 112, 137

athletes, as examples of healthy eating, 184–185

attention deficit disorder (ADD). *See* ADD (attention deficit disorder)

attention deficit hyperactivity disorder (ADHD). *See* ADHD (attention deficit hyperactivity disorder)

Australia, removal of toxic ingredients in food products, 46

autism, 1, 7, 41, 42, 58, 70, 78

autolyzed yeast, 58

avocados, 135, 141, 145, 238

Ayurveda, 143

B

B3 (niacin), 125

B5 (pantothenic acid), 125. *See also* vitamin B5

B6 (folic acid), 125. *See also* vitamin B6

Baby Einstein, 44

baby food, 19, 154

baby formula, 24, 72–73, 194

bacon, 78, 79, 229

bacteria, good compared to bad, 114–115

bad breath, 128

"bad" cholesterol, 68, 70, 128. *See also* LDL cholesterol

bad diet, as killer, 50

bad odors, 128

badgering, not succumbing to, 45, 175

baked goods, 2, 88. *See also specific baked goods*

balanced diet, 1, 3

bananas, 74, 96, 120, 122, 129, 141

banyanbotanicals.com, 143

bargaining, with kids for what they want, 187, 189

basil, 127

beans
  black, 160, 241, 245
  cannellini, 240
  in general, 27, 145
  Great Northern, 240
  green, 8, 19, 99, 127, 146, 165, 170, 194
  as spring food, 145
  white, 240
  white navy, 240

beef hot dog, 100

beef industry, 22, 28, 32

beef jerky, 79

beer, 32, 64

beets, 123, 147

begging, giving in to, 3

behavior modification techniques, 149, 151, 226

behavioral disorders/issues, 43, 107, 135

Bell and Evans (brand), 102

bell peppers
  in general, 98, 146, 180, 229, 246
  green, 127
  mixed colored, 135
  purple, 130
  red, 123
  sweet, 140
  yellow, 120

belly fat, 131

berries
  black raspberries, 130
  blackberries, 130, 146, 220
  blueberries, 130, 131, 132, 146, 230, 232, 237
  chokeberries, 130
  cranberries, 123, 144, 147

brain development, 63–64, 112
brain function, 124
brainwashing, 24, 45, 91
brands
    Amy's, 98–99
    Annie's, 98
    Bell and Evans, 102
    Bragg's, 229, 235
    EO, 115
    Fage, 116
    Johnson & Johnson, 65
    Kashi, 98
    Kraft, 46, 82, 93
    Rainbow Light, 108
    Siggi's, 231
    Stoneyfield Farms, 116, 181, 245
    365 (Whole Foods), 65, 93
    Yakult, 116
bratwurst, 101
bread, 70, 102. *See also* buns,
    hamburger and hot dog; pita bread;
    white bread
bread sticks, 135
breadcrumbs (Japanese panko), 102
breakfast cereals, 53, 56, 77. *See also*
    cereals
breakfasts, 2, 135
breast cancer, 41, 64, 133
breast milk, 27
breath, bad, 128
breath mints, 56
breathing difficulties, 79
broccoli, 6, 27, 33, 44, 60, 99, 126,
    127, 141, 146, 154, 180, 190, 194,
    218
brown rice, 105
brownies, 11
Brussels sprouts, 127, 147, 155
budgetary concerns, for families,
    159–161, 167
budgetary restrictions, of schools, 9
budgets/budgeting, involving
    children in, 161, 225
bulk, buying in, 173
buns, hamburger and hot dog, 93, 94,
    100, 101, 105

burgers. *See* hamburgers
butane, 94, 101
butter lettuces, 236
butterfly release, 12
butternut squash, 120
butters
    cashew, 139
    clarified, 71
    peanut, 2, 18, 32, 139, 174
butylatedhydroxyanisole (BHA/
    BHT), 77–78

C
cabbage, 127, 130, 141
cake, 64, 70, 129
calcium, 24, 26, 27, 40, 57, 121, 128,
    177, 211
calcium absorption, 125, 126, 128,
    131
calcium caseinate, 58
calories
    in average soda serving, 173
    cautions with diet drinks, 56
    in coconut water, 74
    consumed from sugar, 165
    in daily soda consumption, 53
    empty, 93
    growing children need more, 173
    HCFS as number-one source of, 33
    in kids' fast-food meal, 160, 176
    at movies, 158
    and refill trap, 92
    as a result of fewer organized
        meals at home, 48
cancer, 6, 31, 64, 70, 77, 79, 82, 94,
    124, 128, 131, 155, 180. *See also*
    breast cancer; colon cancer; prostate
    cancer
cancer cell growth, 130, 165
cancer-fighting greens, 155
candy, 61
canned soups, 61
canola, 88
canola oil, 37, 38, 39, 88, 101, 102,
    110, 111, 231

cantaloupes, 120, 211
carbon footprint, of one ham
	sandwich, 30
carbonyl, 108
carcinogens, 41, 77, 82
cardiovascular disease, 72
cardiovascular system, 6, 129
caregivers, as part of program in
	eating right, 182
carotenoids, 121
carotinoid, 128
carrots, 27, 76, 98, 120, 129, 145, 153,
	160, 174, 191, 199, 211, 218, 243
casein, 92
cash incentives, to farmers, 76
cashew butter, 139
cashews, 246
cauliflower, 27, 98, 134, 218
cayenne pepper, 144
celery, 18, 127, 140, 218, 246
celery powder/celery juice, 78, 79
cellular damage and repair, 125
Center for Science in the Public
	Interest (CSPI), 82
Center for Veterinary Medicine, 37
cereals
	artificial colors in, 46
	aspartame in, 53, 56
	breakfast cereals, 53, 56, 77
	as "fortified," 86
	label reading, 86, 171
	marketing budget of, 5
	nutritious cereals, 135
	as source of parabens, 64
	sugary cereals, 36, 45, 85, 135, 163,
		203, 224
challenges
	of author around building lifelong
		healthy eating habits, 5
	availability of food, 33
	in avoiding artificial colors and
		flavors, 81
	in being consistent, 187
	in eating out, 28
	in eating seasonally, 142–143, 221

family challenges, 47–48
	as increasing the longer you wait,
		151
	of instilling healthy eating habits,
		1, 43–47, 51, 153–161
	with organic foods, 107
	in restaurants, 91
cheese
	American cheese, 36
	blue cheese, 237
	casein, 92
	and crackers, 23
	dehydrated, 93
	as dip, 99
	in Europe and other countries, 46
	fake cheese, 207
	feta cheese, 241
	goat cheese, 236
	macaroni and cheese (mac n'
		cheese), 2, 93, 99, 107
	Mexican blend, 245
	Monterey jack, 245
	rBST-free, 91, 98
	as winter food, 144
cheese puffs, 90
cheese sticks, 23, 135
Cheetos, 17
chemical substitutes, 58
chemical-free foods, 46
chemicals, in food, 6, 39, 42, 46, 47,
	93, 101, 113, 114, 139, 148, 202.
	See also fakers; food additives;
	herbicides; pesticides; swindlers;
	tricksters; *specific chemicals*
cherries, 82, 95, 123, 140, 144, 145
chestnuts, 144
Chewable Berries (Nordic Naturals),
	108
chewing gum, 77
chicken
	antibiotic-free, 161
	baked, recipe for, 233–234
	fried, homemade, 102
chicken dogs, 100
chicken enchiladas, recipe for, 245

raw foods, 126, 146

real foods. *See* real food

recommended (eat the rainbow), 118–132

salty foods, 1, 6, 44, 91, 95

spring foods, 145

summer foods, 146

trigger foods, 14

white foods, 134

whole foods, 1, 6, 18, 51, 136, 154

winter foods, 144

formaldehyde, 55–56

fortified, compared to enriched, 86

Four-Grain Pancakes Served with Homemade Applesauce (recipe), 231

Fox, Robin, 178

fractures, 25, 26

freak outs, in public, 193

free radicals, 131

French fries, 95, 102–103

fresh food, 85

fried chicken, 102

frisée lettuce, 236

frozen fruit, 118, 129, 132, 181

frozen vegetables, 19, 60, 118, 160, 161, 246

fructose, 72

fruit garden, 222

fruit juice, 36, 80, 96, 135, 150

fruit punch, 95

fruit salad, 129

fruit snacks, 90, 150

fruits

in baby food, 19

blue fruits, 130–132

dried, 80

farm subsidies, 33

frozen, 118, 129, 132, 181

green fruits, 126–129

as healthy breakfast item, 135

least contaminated, examples of, 141

orange fruits, 119–122

perceived costs of, compared to fast-food meal, 159–160

as preferable to fries, 95

purple fruits, 130–132

red fruits, 123–126

SKU numbers, 17

toxins on outer skins of, 132

white fruits, 133–134

year-round access to, cautions with, 148

yellow fruits, 119–122

fullness, 208

fullyraw.com, 126

"Fun" food, 150, 171–172

G

Gabrielle White Bean Chicken Stew (recipe), 240

gallbladder, 155

games

about food choices, 211–213

computer games, 13

at mealtimes, 209, 210, 211–212

video games, 6

Gandhi, 1

gardens

fruit, 222

herb garden, 220

mini garden, 117

organic, 9, 195

vegetable, 219–220, 222

garlic, 134, 144

gastroesophageal reflux disease (GERD), 24

gastrointestinal system, 6

gelatin, 58

generation test, 172

genetically engineered (GE) foods, 37

genetically modified (GM) foods, 2, 21, 28, 32, 35, 36–39, 46, 51, 66, 70, 76, 87, 88, 95, 102, 110, 138, 172. *See also* GM soy

genetically modified (GM) potatoes, 95, 138

genetically modified organism (GMO), 36, 38

GERD (gastroesophageal reflux disease), 24

German sausage, 101
gestational diabetes, 41
ghee, 71, 229, 238, 240, 243
"Ghee is life" (Sarva Darsana
  Sangraha), 71
ghrelin (hunger hormone), 72
Girl Scouts, 197
glucose, 72
glutamic acid, 58
gluten, 12, 32, 92, 105–106, 109, 135,
  185
gluten-free, 102
GM (genetically modified) foods. See
  genetically modified (GM) foods
GM soy, 37, 66, 70, 88, 95, 102, 110
GMO (genetically modified
  organism), 36, 38
goat cheese, 236
goat milk, 27
Gomasio Seaweed Salt, 62
good bacteria, compared to bad
  bacteria, 114–115
"good" cholesterol, 68, 70, 128
good food, differentiating from junk
  food, 35
"GoodPop" frozen pops, 181
gout, 126
governments
  foreign, banning importation of
    certain US foods, 46
  foreign, removing toxic
    ingredients in food products, 21,
    46–47
  responsiveness of to parents/
    community concerns, 9
  US, FDA (Food and Drug
    Administration). See FDA (Food
    and Drug Administration)
  US, food subsidies/farm subsidies,
    31–34
grains, 1, 98, 105, 134, 135
grape juice, 80
grape tomatoes, 138
grapefruit, 123, 143, 144
grapes, 123, 127, 130, 132, 140, 147,
  181

Great Northern beans, 240
Greek yogurt, 85, 116, 135, 181, 245,
  248
green beans, 8, 19, 99, 127, 146, 165,
  170, 194
Green Chile Chicken Enchiladas
  (recipe), 160, 245
green fruits, 126–129
green leafy salad, 99
green leafy vegetables, 111
green lettuce, 126, 127
green onions, 127
green peas, 155, 205
green vegetables, 126–129, 153–155
green-light foods, 212
greens, 140, 145, 155. See also collard
  greens
grenadine, 95
grilled, as preferable to fried, 95
grocery budget. See budgetary
  concerns
grocery stores. See also specific stores
  ad campaigns at, 22
  center aisles of, 85
  compared to fast food, 34
  foods to avoid when shopping, 52
  lack of (food deserts), 33
  pester and persistence factors of,
    187
  as platform for teaching nutrition,
    225
  produce selections, 223
  saving money at, 137
  shopping with kids, 224–225
  stick to periphery/perimeter of,
    171, 224
  you are the boss at, 225
ground rules, 182
"grow food," 156, 197
growing pains, 126
growth hormones, 28, 35, 186
guacamole, 135
guava, 120
guidelines, 177
gum, chewing, 77

impact on good bacteria, 115
parabens as mimicking estrogen,
64
hot chocolate mix, 56
hot dogs, 2, 15, 19, 28, 36, 46, 61, 78,
79, 94, 100–101
hot lunch, at school, 8
hot sauce, 138
hummus, 157, 174, 212
Huntington's disease, 59
hydrogenated oil, 95, 101
hydrolyzed protein, 58, 60
Hyman, Mark, 42, 139, 186, 254, 256,
261
hyperactivity, 13, 59, 81, 82, 83, 107,
165

I

ice cream, 3, 70, 90, 181, 194
iceberg lettuce, 137, 155
ice-cream sandwiches, mini, 181
iced tea, 96
ICEE (frozen carbonated beverage),
157
illnesses. *See specific illnesses*
immune dysregulation, 115
immune system, 6, 81, 112, 113, 121,
125, 126, 128, 130, 133, 148, 155
incentives, cash, to farmers, 76
Indika (restaurant), 236
indulgences, by caregivers, 182
industrialized agriculture, 20. *See also*
agricultural companies; big food
companies
inflammation, 24, 63, 70, 111, 112,
125, 186
ingredients
excessive number of in non-
recommended foods, 18, 52, 66,
85, 94, 148, 172, 204
synthetic, 101
inhalation toxicity, 115
instant gratification, 194
insulin, 97, 108, 186
Integrative Nutrition (Rosenthal), 147,
257, 262

iodine, 62, 126
IQ, 107, 216
iron, 62, 108, 128, 129
iron absorption, 121, 125, 128
"it's ok to be sneaky" mentality, 184
IZZE Sparkling Juice, 90

J

Japanese breadcrumbs (panko), 102
jelly, 64
Johnson & Johnson (brand), 65
Journal of Applied Technology, 64
*Journal of Epidemiology and
Community Health*, 216
Joy of Cooking, 231
joyfulbelly.com, 143
juices. *See also specific juices*
alternative to, 229
as dessert option, 104
fruit juice, 36, 80, 96, 135, 150
in general, 73, 103
pure, 75
junk food
and acne, 186
commercials on TV, 203
costs of, 33
determination of moms to avoid,
52
differentiated from good food, 35,
52
effects of, 6
as everywhere, 156–158, 195
and farm subsidies, 32
impacts of, 72, 135
just say "no" to, 157–158
masquerading as real food, 32–36
national bad habit, 1, 8
no such thing, 139
as not filling, 122
not giving in to requests for, 225
parents' belief that junk food is
healthy option, 3
pervasiveness of, 156
placating and rewarding with, 4
in school vending machines, 9

sugar content of, 163
talking to kids about dangers of, 49
junk food addiction cycle, breaking of, 157–158, 166
junk-food masqueraders, 32–33
just say "no," to junk food, 157–158, 225

K

kale, 27, 126, 127, 144, 155, 205, 211, 230
Kashi (brand), 98
kashi.com, 98
kefir yogurts, 116
ketchup, 36, 93, 94, 95, 100, 102, 138
kids' menus at restaurants, 3, 19, 91–96, 180
kidskeeptheearthcool.org, 31
kielbasa, 101
KISS (Keep It Simple Stupid), 216
kitchen
    as gathering place, 206
    kids helping out in, 214–216
kiwi, 127, 141
kolaches, 2, 135
kosher hot dogs, 100
Kraft (brand), 46, 82, 93
krill oil, 67, 112, 113
Kristina (at fullyraw.com), 126

L

label-reading guidelines, 84–90
labels
    as deceptive, 60, 84, 148
    decoding, 84–90
    on European products, 46
    need for on GM foods, 21, 36, 37, 138
    on non-GMO foods, 87
    reading and studying of, 18, 37, 38, 52, 65, 84–90, 108, 135, 171, 172, 203, 226
lactic acid, 93
lactose, 93

lactose intolerance, 25
Lambert, Beth, 114
Last Child in the Woods (Louv), 13
laws of the house, 168–171
LDL cholesterol, 133. *See also* "bad" cholesterol
lead, 78
lean meats, 1
lecithin, 2
leeks, 144
lemon juice, 80
lemonade, 75, 95, 96, 229
lemons, 103, 144
lettuce
    butter, 236
    on fast-food sandwiches, 17, 174
    frisée, 236
    green, 126, 127
    iceberg, 137, 155
    as one of most contaminated vegetables, 140
    red-tipped, 123, 238
    romaine, 155
    spring, 145, 155
Lew, Gary, 150
Lick the Sugar Habit (Appleton), 165
life skills, development of, 214
lifestyle change, 204
Light and Crisp Citrus Dressing (recipe), 237
lime juice, 80
limes, 103, 127
"liquid candy" (soft drinks), 170
liquid dietary food supplements, 64
Little Smokies, 78
Little Sugar Addicts (DesMaisons), 165, 261
Live Well Network, 160
liver (body organ), 115, 128, 155
longevity, 6, 21, 52
Lou Gehrig's disease (ALS), 53–54, 59
Louv, Richard, 12–13
loveandlogic.com, 190, 192, 194
lunch
    balanced, 100

CPSIA information can be obtained at www.ICGtesting.com
Printed in the USA
LVOW121403180113

316308LV00012B/114/P